mother and baby
NATURAL CARE

French WELLNESS SECRETS AND RECIPES
FOR NEW AND EXPECTING MOTHERS
AND THEIR LITTLE ONES

**WELLBEING ADVICE BY
NATURALIST MIDWIFE HÉLÈNE BOYÉ**

**PHOTOGRAPHY, STYLING, TEXT,
AND RECIPES BY ÉMILIE HÉBERT**

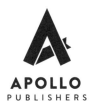

APOLLO
PUBLISHERS

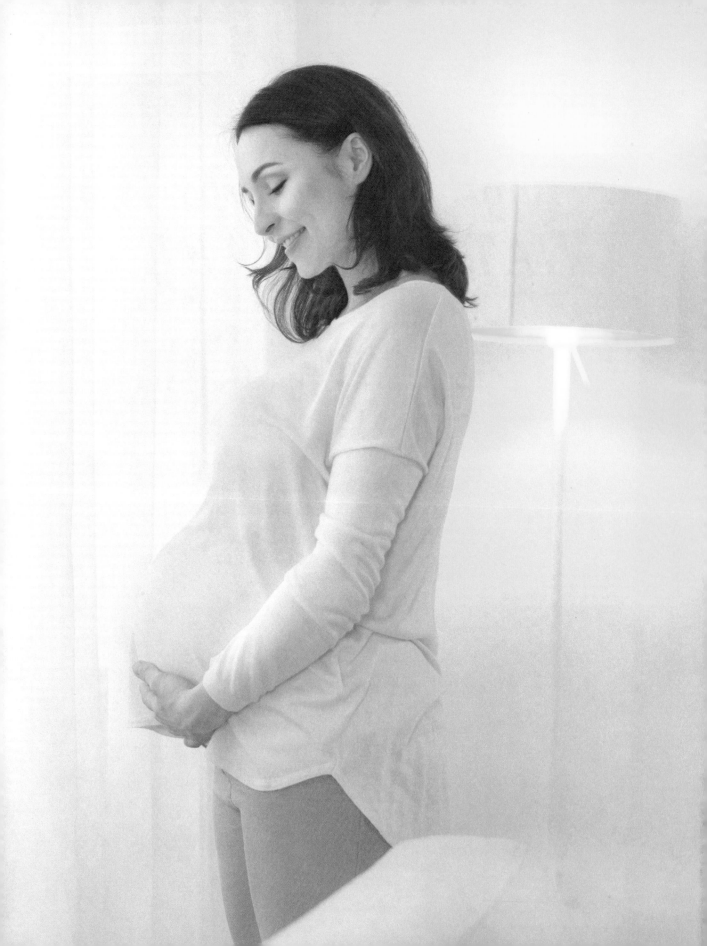

PREFACE

〜〜〜〜〜

Having worked as a midwife for more than twenty years, I have always tried to look at pregnancy, childbirth, and post-childbirth from a physiological standpoint—and by this I mean with an understanding of how the body normally functions. To me, it is essential to teach mothers-to-be how their bodies function during these different processes, and especially what resources a mother has while experiencing them, in order to prepare her for the delivery and birth of the baby.

Western medicine has an unfortunate tendency to divide up the body and its functions. The uterus belongs to one category, the baby's development another, and the bony pelvis and posture to yet another . . . without any acknowledgment of how they are all connected.

During my various travels as a midwife for Doctors Without Borders, I discovered Chinese medicine through acupuncture, which I have now been practicing for fifteen years. It has allowed me to listen to and provide holistic support to future mothers so they can reconnect with their own resources and have positive experiences of these essential life events.

By becoming aware that the body and the spirit form a whole, a woman can reclaim her pregnancy, the birth itself, and her role as a mother. Assuming agency during pregnancy, birth, and our entire lives naturally leads us on the path to more conscious, ethical, and sustainable behavior in terms of our eating habits, personal hygiene, and self-care.

Émilie Hébert's recipes will be invaluable for all mothers who want to take control of their bodies and take care of themselves and their babies in a healthy, responsible way. Let's discover the benefits of what nature offers us and the joy of making healthy, effective products ourselves!

Hélène Boyé

WARNING

All content contained in this book is purely informative and can in no way be considered as a medical prescription or a replacement for advice from your doctor or your child's doctor. Consult with medical professionals prior to usage.

CONTENTS

~~~~~~~~~

TREATMENTS FOR MOM

TREATMENTS FOR BABY

WHAT IS A NATURAL AND ORGANIC PRODUCT?

~~~~~~~~

Have you ever wondered what a conventional beauty product contains? Questionable ingredients, chemical preservatives, endocrine disruptors, and other carcinogenic ingredients . . . the list goes on.

Beauty products that are certified organic are meant to be nontoxic. They have natural raw materials, they are biodegradable, and they are not tested on animals. Their composition excludes any controversial ingredients.

There is no official standard for products that are designated as "green" or "natural," whereas the term "organic" is a label that ensures compliance with a well-defined charter.

Any manufacturer can claim that their beauty product is "natural" just because they have added 0.1 percent organic lavender essential oil in a formulation that is otherwise 99.9 percent artificial. So beware of product packaging: a cute chubby baby, a pretty flower, a field of wheat, or an understated, pharmaceutical-type label does not reflect a truly natural composition. Only the INCI[1] will tell you exactly what the product you're holding in your hands contains.

DECIPHERING LABELS

It can be quite difficult for ordinary people to decipher the labels of beauty products, which are not designed to be read by the average person. However, given the contradictory studies on the possible toxicity of certain substances, it is a good idea to look up a cosmetic's ingredients by referring to the INCI

designation (see page 17). Please note that the ingredients indicated in the composition for beauty products are displayed in descending order of concentration. This means that the first four or five ingredients in the INCI list make up the greater part of the product.

FINDING THE LABELS

The best way to be certain about what you're getting is to choose products that have labels. The "organic" label guarantees that there are no ingredients that could be toxic to you or your baby. In France, there are different labels: "Nature" (with three degrees of certification: natural beauty products, natural and organic beauty products, and organic beauty products), Cosmébio d'Écocert, Nature & Progrès, Soil Association (for products from Great Britain), BDIH (for German products), and ICEA (for Italian products). There are others, but these are the most common. The "AB" ("agriculture biologique") label, on the other hand, is for food. Some food products, such as vegetable oils or essential oils, that are used in the production of home beauty products may have this logo.

It is worth learning how to spot the symbols for these labels and also to identify those that have nothing to do with any certification and therefore offer no guarantee; they were simply made up to emphasize one detail about a product without offering any guarantee regarding the rest of its composition. It's marketing, pure and simple! For this reason, you have to know how to read between the lines.

~~~~~~~~

1 International Nomenclature of Cosmetic Ingredients—this is the list of ingredients that a cosmetic product contains.

Some organic products like shower gels and shampoos certainly cost more, but their environmentally-friendly manufacturing process and plant-based raw materials mean they are high-quality and safe. Nature provides us with a diverse range of ingredients that are too-often neglected in favor of synthetic substances of questionable safety, especially for mothers-to-be and newborns. The best way to make sure that your beauty products are safe is to make them yourself, with natural raw materials, even from your own garden!

CHOOSE YOUR INGREDIENTS WELL

Organic beauty products are nontoxic, paraben-free, and silicone-free. They are biodegradable and not tested on animals. Their raw materials come from organic farming, so they don't contain pesticides or chemical fertilizers. Synthetic ingredients are sometimes found in organic beauty products—they are used to preserve, to create foam—but don't worry, controversial raw materials are not allowed.

Conventional beauty products contain active ingredients at concentrations of 0.01 percent, chemical preservatives, synthetic oils derived from petrochemicals, and substances that may be allergenic, irritating, or even carcinogenic. On the other hand, organic beauty products offer quality care based on active ingredients and are free of chemical and polluting substances which, in the long term, are harmful to our bodies and the environment.

Contrary to popular belief, organic beauty products are not necessarily more expensive. But is a safe organic product really comparable to a conventional beauty product that is made primarily of paraffin oil and water, anyway? And when we compare them with luxury brands, which do not necessarily have better ingredients, organic beauty products clearly have the advantage in terms of price. The cost of advertising and packaging is passed on to the customers!

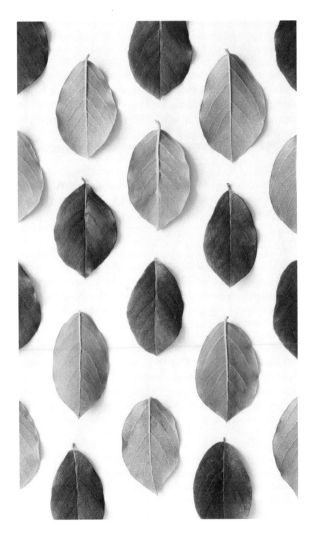

WHY GO NATURAL WHILE PREGNANT?

~~~~~~~~~~

Pregnancy is a time when everything changes! And, like a revelation, it becomes clear that going natural is the solution. You've chosen to turn to more natural products that are safe and environmentally friendly in order to help your body cope with the shifts that pregnancy can cause: to nourish your skin, massage your muscles, prevent stretch marks, activate blood circulation, and also to pamper yourself!

Pregnancy is an important stage—it's a pivotal time in a woman's life. A woman's desire to listen to her own body and instincts often comes naturally, and she'll want to use the healthiest and most natural things for herself and her unborn child. During this period, our bodies change and so do our states of mind!

When a woman is pregnant, certain toxic molecules can enter the blood of the mother-to-be and cross the placental barrier. During organogenesis,[2] this can cause permanent fetal malformations. Of these toxic substances, endocrine disruptors are your number-one enemy. Yet they are prevalent in beauty products, food, bottles, toys, clothes, bed linens, and even on walls (in paint)! According to the World Health Organization (WHO) and the United Nations Environment Programme (UNEP), endocrine disruptors are a real threat to our health and our babies' health. Therefore, when you are pregnant, avoid beauty products with components that can pose risks to the fetus, especially those that pass the skin barrier such as endocrine disruptors, parabens, phthalates,

and nanoparticles (which are present, for example, in makeup and sunscreen products; see pages 16 and 17) as much as you can.

However, beware that certain essential oils with neurotoxic and abortifacient molecules are off-limits for pregnant women (see pages 30 and 31). Active cosmetic ingredients derived from essential oils or plant extracts, particularly supercritical CO_2 extracts, should also be handled with care. Retinol (provitamin A), reputed to be toxic to the fetus, is also to be avoided.

WHAT IS THE COCKTAIL EFFECT?

Conventional commercial products are not dangerous if used sporadically. But the regular accumulation of potentially harmful substances creates a "cocktail effect" in our bodies.

Substances that are not theoretically toxic on their own and in minute doses can, however, become dangerous when they accumulate or mix with other substances. Safety tests are only performed on one product at a time and not on several products used simultaneously (day cream + serum + foundation + shower gel + shampoo, etc.). According to a study

~~~~~~~~~~

2   This is the crucial period of organ formation in the fetus; it lasts about three months.

conducted by Yves Rocher, European women apply approximately nine pounds of beauty products, including makeup, to their faces each year. Just imagine the amount of potentially harmful ingredients that accumulate every day in our bodies!

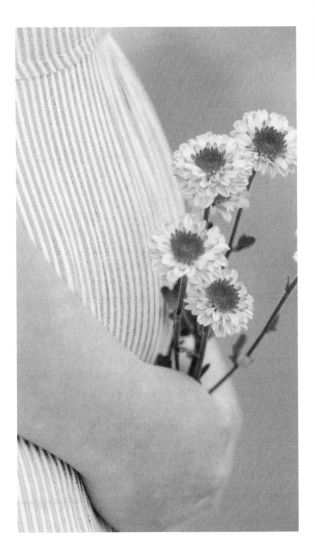

GOOD HABITS FOR FUTURE MOTHERS

❋ *Invest in products specially formulated for pregnant women.*

❋ *Give preference to products with an organic label.*

❋ *Opt for vegetable oils: they nourish and soften the skin, soothe itching, prevent stretch marks, and even reduce the pregnancy mask (see page 41)—without any risk.*

PHTHALATES: DANGEROUS FOR PREGNANT WOMEN

Phthalates are chemicals that can cross the placenta and are toxic to the fetus. A US study has linked them to changes in the level of thyroid hormones, which are essential for brain development. In addition, they affect the neurons linked to the development of motor skills. Previous research has established a link with other disorders, particularly of boys' reproductive systems and behaviors.

WHY CHOOSE NATURAL PRODUCTS FOR YOUR BABY?

Baby has arrived! This tiny person is undoubtedly the greatest motivation to adopt a more natural lifestyle. Newborns have fragile and reactive skin, yet most products designed for them contain high percentages of synthetic materials. Ensuring the purity and quality of the products you use for them also means protecting them!

THE LIVER IS IMMATURE

In infants the liver is still immature and does not produce all the enzymes needed to eliminate foreign molecules that accumulate in the body, meaning there are risks of toxicity. It is estimated that the liver reaches maturity around five or six years of age. During breastfeeding, foreign molecules can pass into the mother's bloodstream and be passed on to the baby through breast milk.

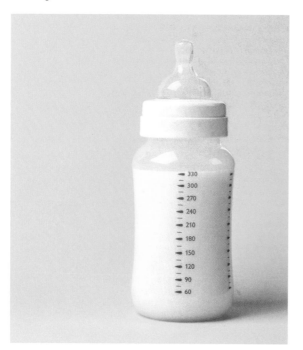

THE RISKS ARE HIGHER IN INFANTS

An infant's skin has normal permeability; a product does not penetrate it any more than it does an adult's skin. Nevertheless, an infant's skin-to-weight ratio[3] brings along an increased risk of being contaminated with toxic substances. However, several studies have shown that a large majority of baby products contain controversial substances.

A study conducted by the nonprofit Women Engage for a Common Future found 299 compounds with ingredients classified as "high risk" or "moderate risk" in 181 of the 341 products tested. This suggests that more than half of the baby products on the market contain substances that are irritating, allergenic, or even hazardous to the baby's health. Similarly, an analysis conducted in October 2013 by the French magazine *Que choisir* showed that more than nine out of ten packages of baby wipes contain endocrine disruptors, allergens, phenoxyethanol, parabens, and the like.

3   An infant's cutaneous surface area is very high in relation to his or her weight.

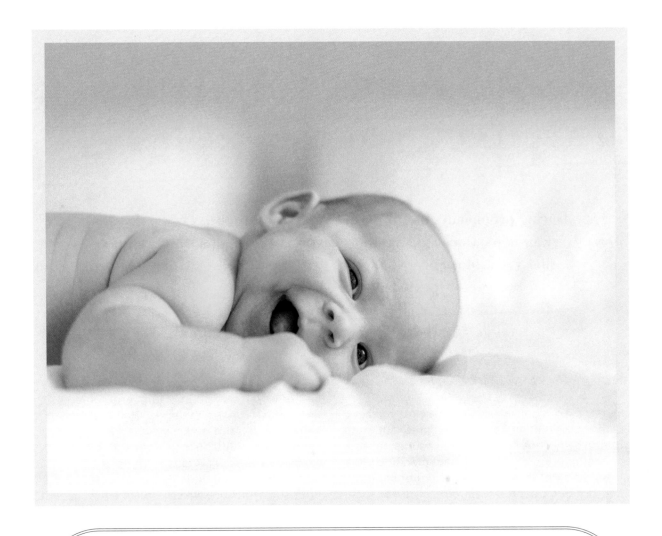

GOOD HABITS FOR BABY

❋ *Focus on the bare minimum. Baby doesn't need a vanity with dozens and dozens of products.*

❋ *Opt for raw materials or beauty products with just a few ingredients, if possible with an organic label.*

❋ *Avoid cleaning wipes as much as possible. If you still want to use them, make sure they do not contain phenoxyethanol, parabens, or perfume.*

TOP INGREDIENTS
TO CHOOSE FROM

~~~~~~~

During pregnancy, the body of the mother-to-be, especially her skin, is particularly stressed. Given the hormonal fluctuations that cause cosmetic changes and weight gain, it is important to use gentle, perfectly-suited care products. This is also the case for the infant, who needs raw products that are as natural as possible. These are safe, healthy, and effective.

ORGANIC VEGETABLE OILS

Vegetable oils are an excellent base for cosmetic care for the mother-to-be during pregnancy and for the baby once born. They are nourishing and, in addition to preventing stretch marks, soothe irritated skin. It is important to choose virgin and organic oils, if possible. This is because, like sugar and flour, conventional vegetable oils undergo a refining process that allows for increased production and longer storage. Through this process, they become inert fats that lose many of their properties. In organic farming, vegetable oils are obtained through mechanical processes whereby they remain cold (or become only very slightly heated). They are produced from mature seeds that have been cultivated using organic methods that respect the environment. They retain all their precious active ingredients: polyunsaturated fatty acids, vitamins, and minerals.

AROMATIC HYDROSOLS

An aromatic hydrosol (sometimes called floral water) is a fresh plant water. Pure or diluted,

it can be used as a facial lotion or as a very gentle treatment for certain problems. It is obtained from the steam of flowers, leaves, twigs, zests, and so on as they are distilled for the production of essential oils. This precious water is filled with the plant's active ingredients and is ideal for natural skin care. Aromatic hydrosols, which contain a tiny amount of the plant's essential oil, are permitted for personal care during pregnancy, but should not be used orally.

VEGETABLE BUTTERS

Vegetable butters are another preferred raw material for use during and after pregnancy. They are rich in active ingredients, very nourishing, anti-inflammatory and antioxidant, and they soften and protect the skin. They are perfect for both mom and baby's skin.

CLAY

Clay is an earthy sedimentary rock that can be used alone or mixed with other ingredients such as vegetable oil, water, or yogurt. It purifies, cleanses, tones, and heals thanks to its aluminum silicate content, and it softens all skin types. Easy to use and inexpensive, clay has been valued as a raw ingredient for thousands of years.

ALOE VERA

Aloe vera is a succulent plant with thick leaves. The gel that is extracted from it has many properties: it's an antiseptic, anti-inflammatory, hemostatic, fungicide, bactericide, and more. It supports the healing of wounds, regenerates cells, and rehydrates and nourishes dry skin. It is used in particular to treat burns, sunburn, irritation, eczema, and chapped skin, but also to help keep the skin from aging. It is very easy to find in pharmacies or health food stores, in a gel form for skin application. But be careful: this gel is often diluted or saturated with synthetic preservatives. Choose as pure a gel as possible (at least 90 percent aloe vera) and preferably certified organic.

NATURAL WAXES

Obtained from plants (carnauba wax, candelilla, etc.) or beeswax, they can thicken cosmetic formulations and have protective film-forming properties that prevent dehydration.

ESSENTIAL OILS

See pages 29 to 33.

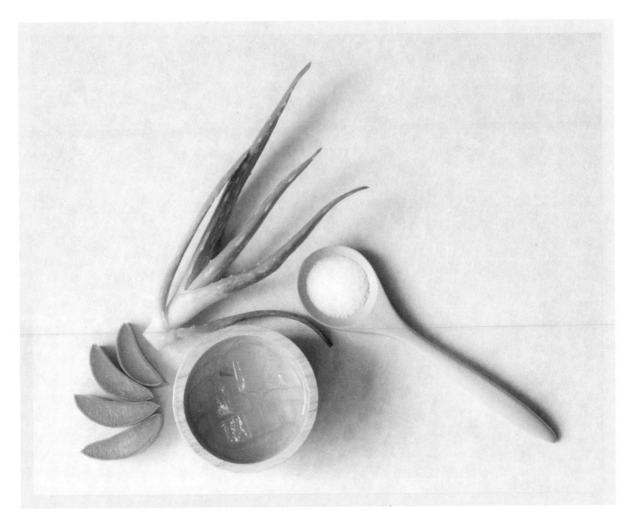

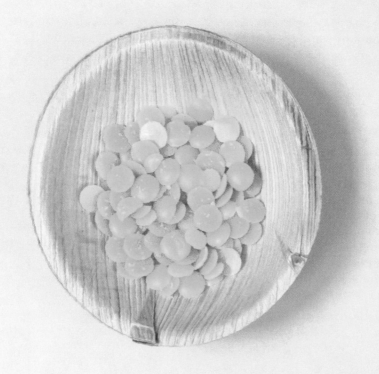

Natural waxes

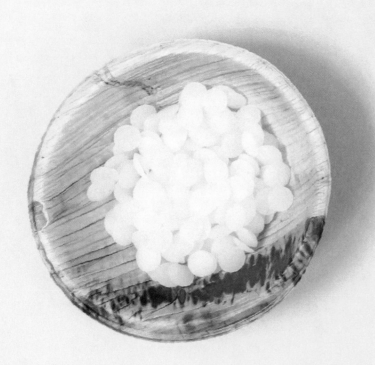

Vegetable oils

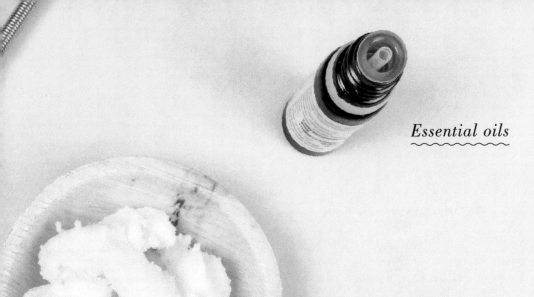

Essential oils

Vegetable butters

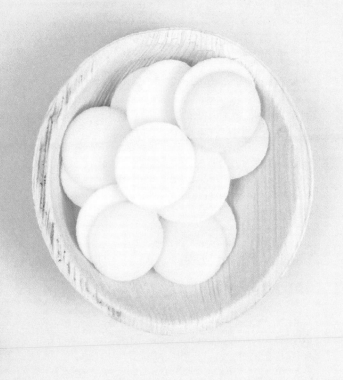

Aromatic hydrosols

TOP INGREDIENTS TO AVOID

MINERAL OILS AND HYDROCARBONS

These are certain alcohols (with the suffix "-anol" in the INCI names: isopropanol, methanol, butanol, ethanol) as well as petrochemical oils like paraffin and petroleum jelly (INCI: paraffinum liquidum, petrolatum, microcrystalline cera, mineral oil, etc.). They clog the pores of the skin and can accumulate in the body, especially in the lymph nodes and liver. They can cause inflammatory reactions, and it is not known what the exact consequences of these are. Some of these substances are even carcinogenic.

SILICONES AND QUATS

According to the INCI nomenclature, silicones have the suffix "-cone" or "-xane" and quats have the suffix "-monium." They are environmentally harmful and also occlusive, meaning they prevent the skin and hair from breathing. They are found almost everywhere, but especially in makeup and hair care. Cyclopentasiloxane and cyclotetrasiloxane are proven endocrine disruptors. In addition, cyclotetrasiloxane is harmful to reproduction.

BHA AND BHT

BHA (INCI: butylhydroxyanisole) and BHT (INCI: butylhydroxytoluene) are allergenic and carcinogenic, according to the International Agency for Research on Cancer (IARC). In addition, they are likely endocrine disruptors, harmful to reproduction.

DEA, MEA, AND TEA

These are found in lotions, sun creams, soaps, shampoos, nail polishes, and more. They are suspected to be carcinogenic (in the liver and kidneys). They are already banned in several countries.

PHENOXYETHANOL

The French National Agency for the Safety of Medicines and Health Products (ANSM) considers phenoxyethanol to be both hematotoxic and hepatotoxic (toxic to the blood and liver). The agency has set limits for children under three years of age. It is unfortunately still present in baby care products or replaced by MIT (see below).

METHYLISOTHIAZOLINONE (MIT)

MIT is the official replacement for the notorious parabens (see opposite). It has been confirmed that this product causes severe allergies.

PROPYLENE GLYCOL AND POLYETHYLENE GLYCOL

These are present in almost all conventional beauty products. An incident of acute poisoning from propylene glycol in a two-year-old child highlighted the potential toxicity of this chemical agent.

TRICLOSAN

This is found in toothpastes and deodorants. This chlorophenol, which has powerful antibacterial and antifungal properties, is a carcinogenic endocrine disruptor. It is believed to affect not just estrogen hormones, but also thyroid function.

SYNTHETIC COLORS

Synthetic colors are found in most beauty products and makeup, and can also be found in hair dye. Animal studies have shown that almost all of them are carcinogenic.

RESORCINOL

This is a colorant, also known as resorcin, used widely in hair dyes. It is highly likely to trigger allergic reactions and should be avoided by those with high sensitivity. But this is not its only shortcoming, as in vivo research has shown that it is an endocrine disruptor.

SULFATES

These include sodium coco sulfate, ammonium lauryl sulfate, sodium laureth sulfate, and sodium myreth sulfate. Derived from sulfur, they are irritants and sensitizers. They are found in shower gels, shampoos, soap substitutes, and sometimes face masks and scrubs.

ARTIFICIAL PERFUMES

Called "fragrances" or "perfumes," they are strongly irritating and allergic.

PARABENS AND OTHER PRESERVATIVES

Parabens, organohalogen compounds (this includes chlorine, bromine, or iodine) and formaldehyde liberators are carcinogenic.

THE INCI AT A GLANCE

❉ *INCI stands for "International Nomenclature of Cosmetic Ingredients," or, in French, "Nomenclature Internationale des Ingredients Cosmetiques." This is a classification system established at the international level in order to have terms that are common to all countries.*

❉ *Ingredients are indicated in English, along with the Latin names for any plants. They are classified in descending order of weight: the closer the ingredient is to the top of the list, the greater the quantity present.*

❉ *Generally speaking, the first four ingredients are considered to make up 90 percent of the end product.*

8 RULES TO FOLLOW TO MAKE YOUR OWN NATURAL CARE PRODUCTS

1 Choose quality ingredients and raw materials. Check the Best By Date (BBD) and keep them stored away from light, heat, and moisture. Make sure the packaging is securely closed following use.

2 It is preferable to use stainless steel or glass utensils (such as Pyrex or borosilicate glass) that can tolerate heat, are easy to sterilize, and don't present any risk of contamination to your homemade beauty care products (heated plastic containers can release toxic compounds such as phthalates or bisphenol A, and these could enter your beauty care products). Avoid metal utensils when handling clays, which absorb aluminum particles and then deposit them onto your skin.

3 Thoroughly sterilize your work surface, equipment, and containers so your beauty products do not get contaminated and so they keep better. Clean them with soapy water and, once they are dry, spray them generously with 70 percent alcohol and allow them to air-dry for a few minutes. Don't wipe the alcohol off—otherwise it won't have enough time to do its job.

4 Keep to the dosages recommended by your suppliers and never substitute one ingredient for another without checking. Dosages and recommendations will vary from one ingredient to another. There may even be interactions between ingredients, so be careful.

5 Label your products with a list of the ingredients used along with their date of manufacture.

6 Do a patch test on your forearm forty-eight hours before using a product to check for any reaction (irritation, redness); the same applies to your child.

7 Use a reliable preservative approved for organic beauty products (such as Cosgard, see page 28), and store your products in a sealed container away from moisture and heat.

8 Put your hair up, close the windows, and make sure pets won't get in the way. Before starting, wash your hands thoroughly and put on a pair of gloves or spray your hands with 70 percent alcohol.

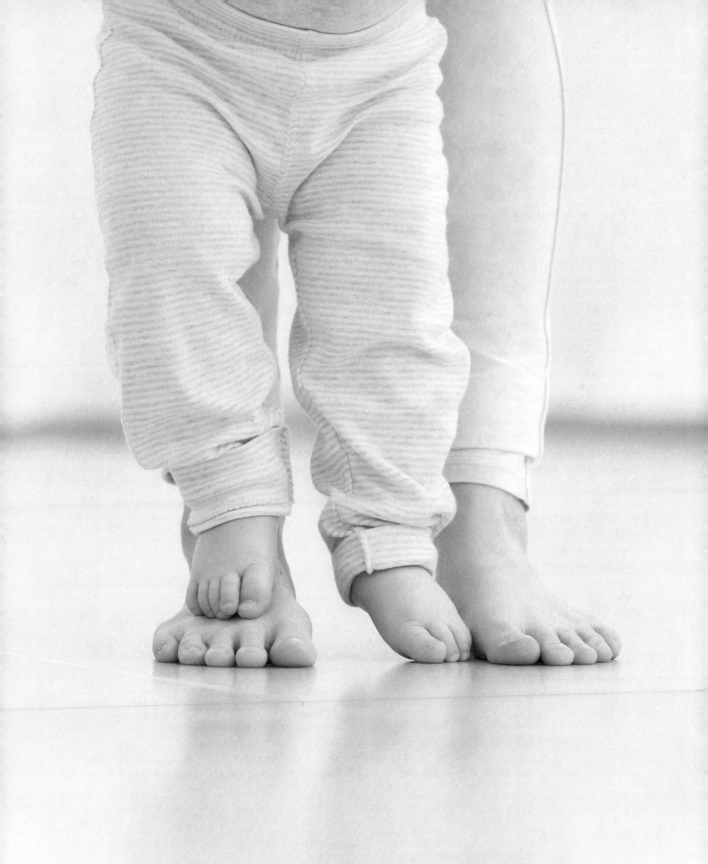

THE IDEAL RAW MATERIALS

PLANT OILS

Sweet almond oil
This is an indispensable oil for mother and baby. It soothes and softens delicate, dry skin. It is used to prepare nourishing care for all—including sensitive—skin types.

Apricot oil
This is a very gentle, softening neutral oil. It gives a healthy glow and is perfect as a base for massage oil or for mother and baby care products.

Avocado oil
Rich in oleic acids (about 60 percent) and phytosterols, avocado oil performs a powerful restructuring action—it stimulates collagen synthesis. It helps to heal wounds, provides intense nourishment to the skin, and helps prevent or reduce stretch marks. It is also rich in palmitic acids (about 20 percent), which are natural components of the skin's protective barrier, and in antioxidant vitamins (C, E, and provitamin A). Avocado oil has excellent properties for face, body, and hair care.

Oat oil
Rich in ceramides and phytosterols, oat oil is soothing, protective, and softening. It is recommended for sensitive, delicate, and reactive skin.

Jojoba oil
This is a very gentle oil with a slightly viscous texture. It moisturizes and soothes dry skin while regulating sebum production in combination and oily skin. It protects the skin from dehydration.

Coconut oil
Virgin coconut oil has a light natural scent. Coconut oil is solid at room temperature and becomes liquid starting at 77°F. Rich in vitamins E, A, and K, it is extremely nourishing. It also has antibacterial properties and is used in natural deodorants and toothpastes.

Raspberry oil
Obtained by cold-pressing raspberry achenes (the small seeds that we notice as we are eating the berries), this oil is rich in vitamin E, polyphenols, and essential fatty acids. It contains very powerful anti-inflammatory agents that calm sensitive and irritated skin. It soothes all types of skin lesions (such as eczema, irritations, and psoriasis). Virgin raspberry oil also has strong anti-UV properties: on its own, it corresponds to an SPF between 30 and 50. It is thus ideal to protect your face from the sun's rays on a daily basis, but it is still no replacement for sun protection.

Tamanu oil
Also known as Calophyllum inophyllum, tamanu helps to strengthen the skin if there is redness, sensitivity, or sagging in the cheeks or sides of the nose. It supports the natural renewal of cells.

MACERATED OILS

Arnica macerated oil
This is ideal for treating aches and bumps and also for reducing bruising, since arnica stimulates blood circulation and is an anti-inflammatory. In addition, this maceration is very useful in reducing stretch marks and soothing sore legs.

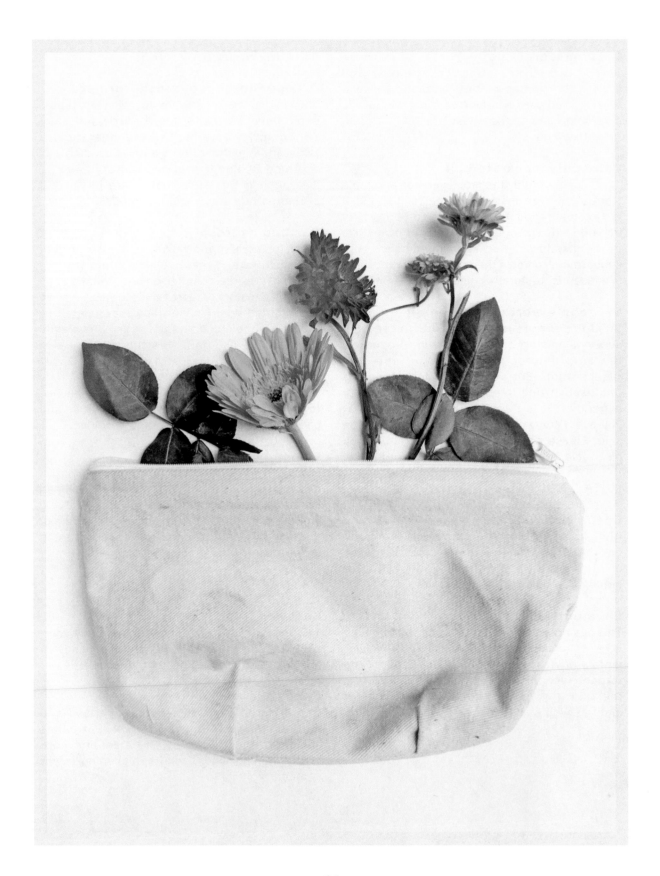

Daisy macerated oil

This is remarkably effective in toning and firming the skin as well as the blood vessels. Widely used particularly in care for the bust to give some pep to the chest, it is ideal during breastfeeding.

Calendula macerated oil

This is undoubtedly the most common and most frequently-used macerate d oil for babies! It is recommended for sensitive, blotchy, and irritated skin. It soothes all kinds of owies like irritations, burns, cracks, chapped hands, and sunburn. It promotes the healing of wounds and is antiseptic, restorative, and anti-inflammatory.

St. John's wort macerated oil

St. John's wort is a plant with incredible anti-inflammatory and pain-relieving properties. It also promotes wound healing and skin regeneration. But beware: St. John's wort is photosensitizing (because of the presence of hypericin). It is therefore recommended that you avoid sun exposure after applying it to the skin. Please note: St. John's wort macerated oil should not be used orally during pregnancy.

PLANT BUTTERS

Cocoa butter

Rich in unsaponifiables and antioxidants, cocoa butter promotes the healing of wounds and is restorative and soothing. It is great for homemade balms and protects dry skin.

Shea butter

This is a nourishing butter that contains a high level of unsaponifiables such as anti-inflammatory phytosterols, antioxidant vitamins, and terpene alcohols that both soften and protect the skin. It is perfect for care products for mom as well as baby.

AROMATIC HYDROSOLS

Orange blossom hydrosol (or neroli)

This hydrosol is suitable for all skin types, especially dry, sensitive, or irritated skin. Soothing, invigorating, and regenerating, it is the ideal hydrosol for gently cleansing and soothing itching, irritation, and erythema. It is especially suited for baby care because it promotes relaxation and sleepiness.

Bamboo hydrosol

Ideal for combination skin, it is also perfect for sensitive and reactive skin. It moisturizes and mattifies the complexion and, thanks to its anti-inflammatory properties, it soothes sensitive and irritated skin. Rich in silica, it remineralizes the skin while stimulating collagen and elastin synthesis. It also promotes cell renewal.

Damascus rose hydrosol

This hydrosol is the beauty water par excellence for all skin types, even sensitive: it firms and soothes the skin while fighting wrinkles.

Lemon hydrosol

Fresh, fragrant, and rich in vitamins, lemon hydrosol refreshes, tones, tightens pores, and promotes a radiant complexion. It is purifying and therefore helps to eliminate imperfections. It is also brightening; it makes your complexion glow and reduces pigmentation spots.

NATURAL WAXES

Beeswax

This is commonly used in mom and baby care, especially in the creation of natural balms. It has film-forming and protective properties.

Candelilla wax

One hundred percent vegetable-derived and natural, this wax is used for making balms and ointments. However, it is harder and more brittle than beeswax, and its thickening power is much higher.

OTHER INGREDIENTS AND AGENTS

Aloe vera gel

This gel is very rich in active ingredients: polysaccharides, enzymes, trace elements, and eighteen amino acids, along with a high number of vitamins (including A, B1, B2, B3, B6, B9, B12, C, and E). Aloe vera gel has very effective applications for the skin. It is moisturizing, antiaging, and firming, but its greatest asset is its ability to aid in the healing of wounds.

White clay

This acts as a magnet for toxins. It eliminates pollutants and impurities and deeply cleanses the skin. Softening and mattifying, it absorbs excess sebum. It is ideal for sensitive skin.

Zinc oxide

This is ideal for the care of sensitive, reactive, or irritated skin. It is a white antiseptic powder that is primarily used to make soothing care products for sensitive skin. Zinc oxide relieves irritation, eczema, and erythema almost instantly.

Bisabolol

This is a natural active ingredient derived from chamomile. Known for its soothing, softening, and repairing properties, it is ideal for sensitive and uncomfortable skin. It is incorporated into balms, oils, and creams.

Vegetable emulsifying wax (Végémulse or Olivem 1000)

Obtained by combining a plant-derived fatty alcohol and acid, these two natural emulsifying waxes make it possible to easily produce all types of emulsions such as creams, milks, and fluids. They promote the creation of liquid crystals that play a role in keeping the skin hydrated.

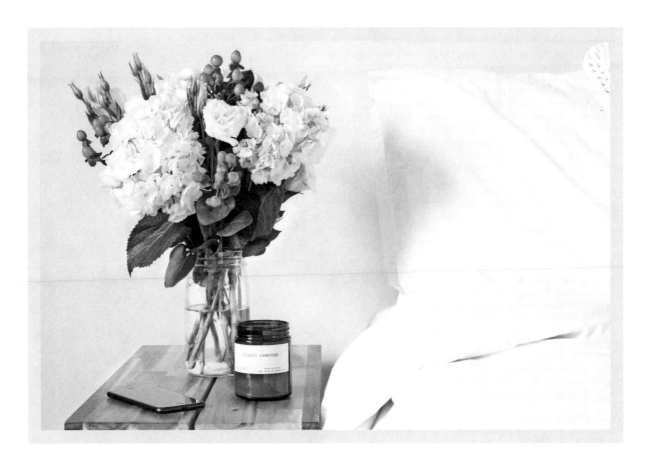

Pink clay
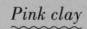

White beeswax
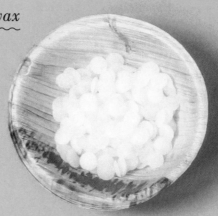

St. John's wort oil
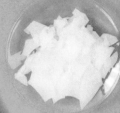

Tamanu oil

Jojoba oil
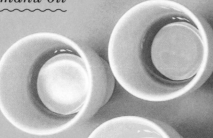

Calendula macerated oil

Emulsifying wax

Zinc oxide

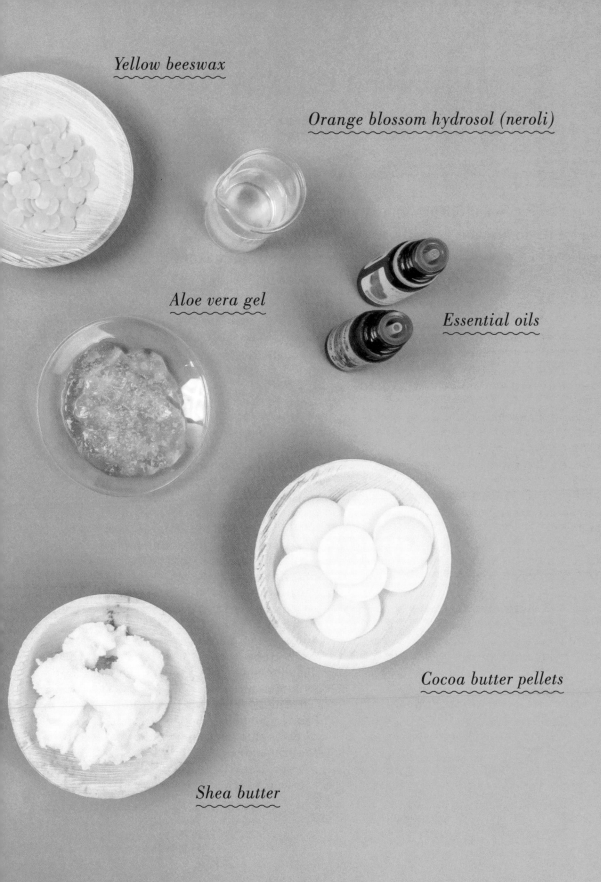

Yellow beeswax

Orange blossom hydrosol (neroli)

Aloe vera gel

Essential oils

Cocoa butter pellets

Shea butter

UTENSILS AND BASIC EQUIPMENT

~~~~~~~~

There's no need to invest in a chemistry set to make your own beauty products. Basic kitchen utensils are more than sufficient for your homemade creations. Of course, you are welcome to invest in beakers or graduated test tubes to make your life easier, but this is by no means a requirement!

BASIC EQUIPMENT

- A kitchen scale
- Several heat-resistant bowls
- A saucepan
- A mortar and pestle
- A manual mini whisk
- A silicone cavity mold (or an ice cube mold)
- A rubber spatula
- 70 percent alcohol for disinfecting (preferably in spray form, for ease of use).

THE LITTLE EXTRAS

(If you want to invest in some more specific utensils.)

- Beakers made of Pyrex or borosilicate glass, or different-sized stainless steel capsules
- An electric mini whisk (cappuccino frother type)
- One small stainless steel (or borosilicate glass) funnel
- A 0.1 g precision scale

PACKAGING

To showcase your products, you can reuse your perfume bottles or glass cream jars. You can also find expensive designer bottles on specialized websites. Garage sales can also be a real gold mine for beautiful old bottles. Reusing is green! Always choose containers that are made of glass, and tinted if possible. Here are a few examples of containers you may need.

- Jars and ointment containers, preferably made of transparent or tinted glass
- Bottles, preferably made of glass, with a spray pump cap
- Recycled jars like glass jelly or jam jars or mason jars for making your macerated oils (see pages 34 and 35)
- Airless pump bottles
- Old perfume bottles (if it has a crimp cap, simply remove it with pliers and replace it with a cork)
- Old, empty cosmetics jars or bottles
- Empty mini jam or honey jars made of glass (the kind found at hotels, for example)

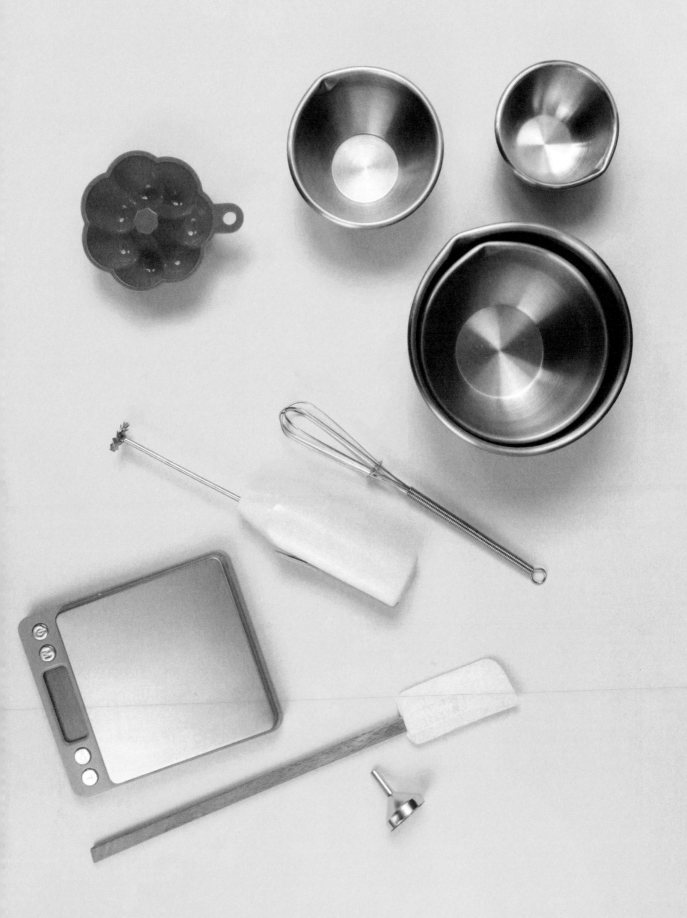

STORING HOME TREATMENTS

To preserve your homemade products, it is necessary to incorporate preservatives, which you can choose depending on the complexity of the formula.

❈ An antimicrobial (like Cosgard) to protect products that contain an aqueous phase (spring water, aloe vera, hydrosol, etc.) from microbes, bacteria, fungi, and yeasts.

❈ An antioxidant (natural vitamin E) to protect fats (oil, butter, wax) from going rancid.

Therefore, a cream (emulsion) containing fats and aqueous bodies will need an antioxidant and an antimicrobial.

An anhydrous (without water) product, such as a balm, will not need antimicrobials in its formula, just as a lotion containing only hydrosols will not need antioxidants.

GOOD HABITS

❈ *Keep your beauty products in a hermetically sealed container.*

❈ *Keep them away from light and heat.*

❈ *Avoid putting your fingers directly into a jar of cream; use a spatula instead.*

	ANHYDROUS PRODUCTS (BALMS, BUTTERS, OILS)	EMULSIONS (CREAMS, MILKS)	AQUEOUS PRODUCTS (LOTIONS, HYDROSOLS)
AVERAGE SHELF LIFE	9 to 12 months	4 to 6 months	3 to 4 months
TYPE OF PRESERVATIVES	Antioxidant	Antimicrobial + antioxidant	Antimicrobial

ESSENTIAL OILS FOR AROMATHERAPY DURING PREGNANCY

Pregnant women are increasingly looking for natural remedies to treat the ailments associated with pregnancy. For this reason, aromatherapy attracts many expectant mothers, but it's important to be very careful with essential oils, as they are not completely risk-free!

During the first three months of pregnancy, they are to be avoided. While it has not been proven that all are harmful to the mother or fetus, some do have proven toxicity. As a precaution, it is therefore advised that they not be used during this crucial period. After the stage of fetal organ formation, only use essential oils that are known to be perfectly safe.

It is important to note that the formulas containing essential oils suggested in this book are only some examples among many. Every expectant mother is to be considered as a unique individual with specific needs.

Unfortunately, alternative medicines are too often abandoned in favor of allopathy (also known as conventional modern medicine), despite the fact that they are gentle and less toxic. This is simply because practitioners do not have sufficient knowledge of natural remedies. However, essential oils offer a veritable natural therapeutic arsenal to midwives.

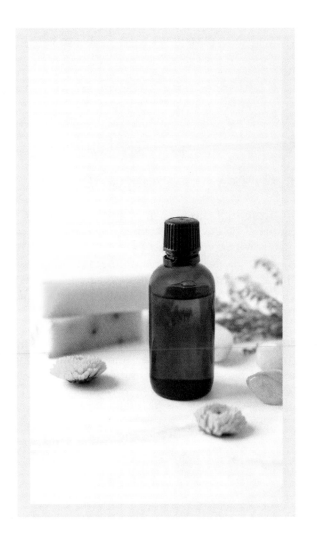

10 GOOD HABITS FOR AROMATHERAPY

1 Rule out the use of all essential oils during the first three months of pregnancy.

2 Also avoid using essential oils until your baby is four months old. Ask your pediatrician for advice if your baby has any allergic conditions.

3 During pregnancy, no essential oils should be taken orally, nasally, ocularly, auricularly, rectally, vaginally, or intravenously without medical advice.

4 Essential oils are effective even at low doses. One drop of essential oil in a tablespoon of vegetable oil or neutral cream is more than enough to be able to benefit from its precious active ingredients.

5 Never use an essential oil you are unfamiliar with without consulting your doctor.

6 Never replace one essential oil with another that you are not absolutely certain is safe.

7 Essential oils are very volatile: close the bottles tightly and place them in a cupboard, away from light and heat (and of course from children!).

8 Only use essential oils for therapeutic uses for specific and occasional needs.

9 Always perform a patch test before applying a product to a large part of the body; some molecules may be allergenic.

10 Avoid sun exposure after using photosensitizing essential oils (especially citrus oils).

WHAT IS AN ESSENTIAL OIL?

An essential oil is an active concentrate of plants (flowers, roots, wood, bark, etc.). It is also sometimes referred to as "quintessential" oil. It is used in beauty products to improve the quality of the skin, but also as a medicinal remedy for the gentle treatment of certain pathologies.

During pregnancy, essential oils are of great help in treating everyday ailments and play a beneficial role in our emotional and overall well-being. They can be precious allies if used wisely.

However, you should be careful and ask your doctor or midwife about any essential oil you wish to use. Unlike fatty vegetable oils, which it is important not to confuse them with, essential oils are volatile. They are made up of aromatic molecules that are indicated by chemotype (we speak of "chemotyped" essential oils or HECT), which serves as a kind of identity card that lets you know what their individual therapeutic properties are and, by extension, the possible risk of toxicity. It is important to check the quality of each essential oil you buy. Its botanical name in Latin must be indicated; it must be chemotyped, 100 percent pure, natural, integral, and, if possible, organic.

ESSENTIAL OILS TO BE AVOIDED DURING PREGNANCY

Natural does not mean harmless! Do not improvise as a practitioner. Essential oils are very powerful. Here is a non-exhaustive list of essential oils that are strictly off-limits for pregnant women, except upon medical advice (CT = chemotype).

Ketone essential oils

In high doses, they are neurotoxic and abortifacient (they can cause miscarriages and result in the loss of the baby). They should be avoided throughout pregnancy.

- Common sage (Salvia officinalis ssp. officinalis)
- Atlas cedar (Cedrus atlantica)
- Camphor rosemary (Rosmarinus officinalis CT camphor)
- Hyssop (Hyssopus officinalis ssp. officinalis)
- Peppermint (Mentha x piperita)
- French lavender (Lavandula stoechas)
- Pennyroyal (Mentha pulegium)

Essential oils with phenols and aromatic aldehydes

Dermocaustic (irritating to the skin) and hepatotoxic (toxic to the liver) at high doses in sensitive individuals, they are to be avoided throughout pregnancy.

- Clove (Eugenia caryophyllus)
- Cinnamon leaves or bark (Cinnamomum verum)
- Cassia cinnamon (Cinnamomum cassia)
- Winter savory (Satureja montana)
- Compact oregano (Origanum vulgare)
- Thyme with thymol (Thymus vulgaris CT thymol)
- Ajwain (Trachyspermum ammi)

Essential oils with geraniol and eugenol

These are uterotonic and can only be used on the day of delivery to help the expectant mother, following professional medical guidance. During the rest of the pregnancy, they are to be avoided.

- Palmarosa (Cymbopogon martinii var. motia)
- Thyme with geraniol (Thymus vulgaris CT geraniol)
- Wild bergamot (Monarda fistulosa)

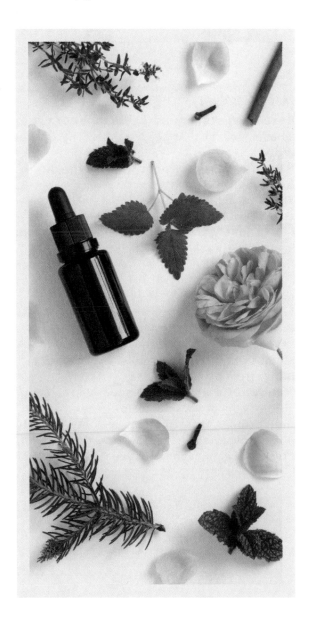

TOP 10 ESSENTIAL OILS FOR MOM AND BABY

In general it is recommended to avoid all essential oils during the first three months of pregnancy. After the first trimester, you can begin to use certain essential oils, especially those composed mainly of monoterpenols, monoterpenes, or esters, without risk to you or your future child.

ROSEWOOD

Botanical Name: Aniba rosaeodora var. amazonica
When?
Mom: from the fourth month of pregnancy
Baby: from six months
Therapeutic properties: mild painkiller, antiseptic, antibacterial, calming, aphrodisiac
Indications: dermatoses, eczema, exhaustion, low morale, feelings of loneliness

NOBLE OR ROMAN CHAMOMILE

Botanical Name: Chamaemelum nobile
When?
Mom: from the fourth month of pregnancy
Baby: from six months
Therapeutic properties: sedative, calming, anti-inflammatory, analgesic
Indications: nausea, stress, anxiety (anxiety during pregnancy, postpartum depression, etc.), eczema, acne, rosacea, sensitive or inflamed skin

LEMON

Botanical Name: Citrus limon
When?
Mom: from the first month of pregnancy
Baby: from six months
Cautions: photosensitizer; avoid sun exposure following application
Therapeutic properties: antibacterial, antiseptic, antiviral, digestive tonic, carminative (reduces gas and facilitates its expulsion), appetite stimulant
Indications: nausea, aerophagia, digestive fatigue, varicose veins, warts, rosacea, hemorrhoids

TRUE LAVENDER

Botanical Name: Lavandula angustifolia
When?
Mom: from the first month of pregnancy
Baby: from six months
Therapeutic properties: antispasmodic, calming, healing, skin regenerating, analgesic, hypotensive, antibacterial
Indications: stress, anxiety, agitation, helps with acceptance of the newborn, softening of the perineum, false contractions, eczema, dermatitis, rosacea

NEROLI

Botanical Name: Citrus aurantium var. amara
When?
Mom: from the fourth month of pregnancy
Baby: from six months
Therapeutic properties: comforting, calming, sedative, promotes a sense of inner peace
Indications: anxiety, stress, sleep disorders; it is the oil for emotional distress

NIAOULI

Botanical name: Melaleuca quinquenervia CT cineole
When?
Mom: from the fourth month of pregnancy
Baby: from six months
Therapeutic properties: powerful antiviral, expectorant, venous decongestant
Indications: weeping eczema, pregnancy mask, water retention, stretch marks, shingles, warts

PALMAROSA

Botanical name: Cymbopogon martinii var. motia
When?
Mom: only on the day of delivery, on medical advice
Baby: do not use for baby.
Therapeutic properties: powerful broad-spectrum antibacterial, antifungal, immune stimulant, uterine and nervous tonic, healing of wounds
Indications: triggering of contractions, strengthening of contractions, facilitating delivery, stress, irritability

SMALL GRAIN BITTER ORANGE

Botanical Name: Citrus aurantium ssp. aurantium
When?
Mom: from the fourth month of pregnancy
Baby: from six months
Therapeutic properties: relaxing, sedative, antidepressant, anti-inflammatory, healing of wounds, skin regenerating
Indications: acne, rosacea, headaches, fear of pain (childbirth), gastric hyperacidity

RAVINTSARA

Botanical Name: Cinnamomum camphora CT cineole
When?
Mom: from the fourth month of pregnancy
Baby: from six months
Cautions: not recommended for asthmatics
Therapeutic properties: antiviral, antibacterial, immunostimulant, expectorant, energizing
Indications: angina, gastroenteritis, flu, insomnia, viral diseases, sore throat

TEA TREE

Botanical Name: Melaleuca alternifolia
When?
Mom: from the fourth month of pregnancy.
Baby: from six months
Therapeutic properties: broad-spectrum antibacterial, antifungal, antiviral, antiparasitic, decongestant
Indications: oral infections, bacterial infections, warts, sore throat, wounds, skin mycoses

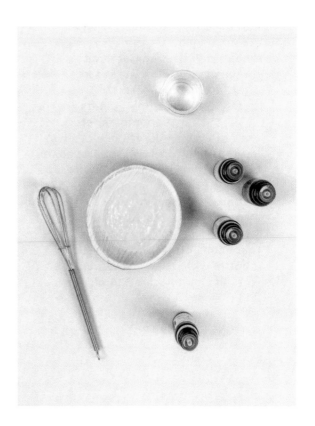

MAKE YOUR OWN MACERATED OILS
FOR MOTHER AND BABY

Oleic extracts, medicinal oils, macerated oils: these oils with beneficial properties go by many names. And there are as many possible macerations as there are plants. Here's how to make them easily and without much expense all on your own.

MATERIALS

❋ A jar with a lid (such as a small Le Parfait jar or recycled glass jam or preserves jar)

❋ A neutral virgin vegetable oil (grapeseed, sunflower, sesame, olive, etc.), preferably organic

❋ High-quality plant ingredients (herbs, flowers, pods, vegetables, etc.), preferably organic, from your own garden, or wild-grown (see opposite)!

❋ A cheesecloth, a sterile compress, a coffee filter, or a very fine strainer—anything that will allow you to filter for a fine, clean macerated oil.

❋ A funnel—not absolutely necessary, but practical!

❋ A bottle with a sealing cap cleaned with alcohol to store the oil, and a label

You can prepare your oils with dried plants (that you've dried yourself or bought in health food stores or from herbalists) or with fresh plants, which work just as well. Note, however, that the plants must not be wet. Otherwise they could alter the preparation and the macerated oil will end up in the trash, which would be a shame! Let the fresh plants lay out for a few hours on a clean and dry cloth, keeping them spaced apart, so that they are not wet when they come into contact with the oil. Turn them over several times if necessary. If in doubt, spread them out on a baking tray and dry them for 1 hour in the oven heated to a maximum temperature of 140°F.

STEP-BY-STEP

1. Fill the jar with plants.

2. Pour in the vegetable oil so that all the plants are submerged. Close the jar tightly.

3. Let the mixture stand in indirect light for four weeks, shaking it from time to time.

4. Filter the mixture gently to collect the oil that is full of the plants' active ingredients.

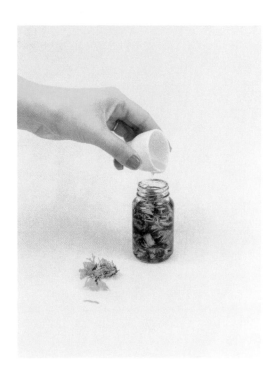

~~~~~~~

GATHERING WILD PLANTS

Before harvesting plants in the wild, it is important to observe the area, be vigilant, and respect the ecosystem. Check that the area is not protected and pick only what you need. Do not uproot plants, or only uproot species of plants that are growing in abundance. Don't pick plants you aren't familiar with, since some of them can be toxic! (You can ask an herbalist after gathering your plants.)

Keep the plants sorted while gathering them and also when preparing the maceration. Also be aware that the younger the plants are, the higher the concentrations they have of active substances.

~~~~~~~

TREATMENTS FOR MOM

DURING PREGNANCY

By Hélène Boyé, naturalist midwife

Pregnancy should be a time of introspection: this body in transformation has the information you need. Pregnancy is not a disease; on the contrary, it is a physiological function. The most important thing is to listen to your own needs, sensations, and feelings: they will always be right.

Expressions like "I don't know why, but I feel that . . ." must be your guides, because then it is not your mind that is speaking; it is your feelings, and they know what is good for you.

Take the time, at least once a week, to reap the benefits of a prenatal yoga session or prenatal water aerobics. Working on breathing, stretching, and postures is essential to better experience the transformation of the body during pregnancy and to prepare for childbirth.

Communication with your baby will be improved by practices centered on your and your partner's senses, like haptonomy (a massage method meant to build an emotional bond between expectant parents and babies before birth) for example. Choose a massage session adapted to your pregnancy in order to feel all the parts of your body; it is an excellent way to care for your body and its tensions.

In self-massage for example, you can take the time every evening to roll a tennis ball under the soles of your feet for five minutes; this stimulates blood circulation and releases tension.

Mindfulness and sophrology (a self-help method popular in Europe that merges Western science and Eastern wisdom) are helpful tools for returning to your breathing and well-being by releasing the mind from the sometimes stressful or anxious thoughts that arise during pregnancy.

TIP: QUICK MORNING MEDITATION

Take a moment to return to your breathing, sitting or lying down in a position that is comfortable for you. Observe how your stomach feels when you breathe in and out: it fills with air when you breathe in and relaxes when you breathe out. Stay there, in the present moment, in touch with the sensations of the breath. If thoughts arise, let them pass without attachment and bring your attention back to the breath coming in and going out of your nostrils. Just be present to what is there . . . the breath . . . your baby's movements . . . your feelings. Remember that pregnancy is a physiological phenomenon, and there's no need to get lost in theory!

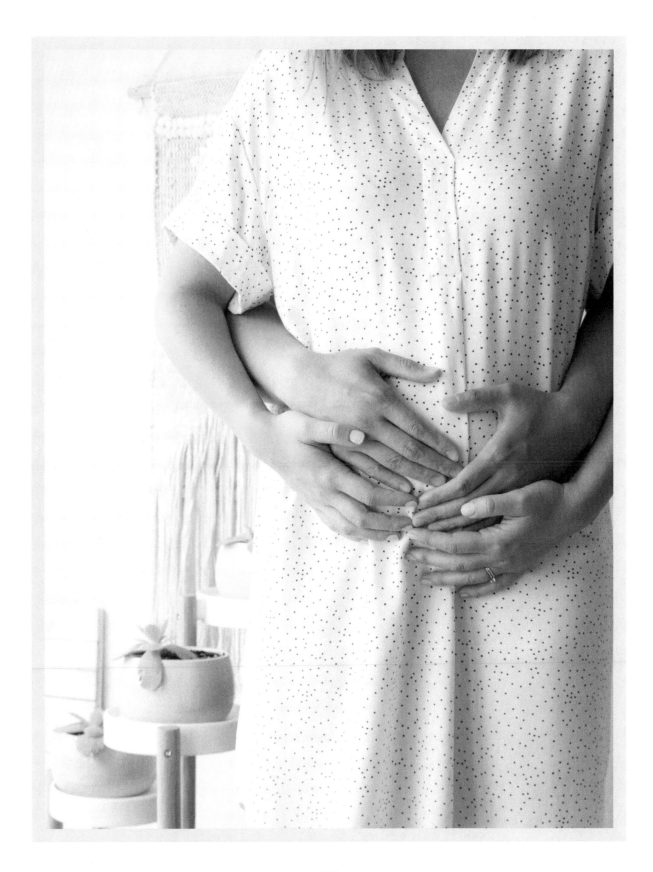

FACIAL TREATMENTS

~~~~

While some women go through their pregnancy with a glow, others will experience problems caused by hormonal changes. Your skin may become more sensitive or more reactive to stressors: this manifests itself through irritations, allergies, itching, tingling, or rosacea. It may even dry out or become greasy. You may see acne appear as a response to the hormonal upheaval that is taking place inside of you. Don't worry! There are some simple steps you can take to preserve your skin and be a radiant mother-to-be!

~~~~

GOOD HABITS

※ *Choose natural products that have the simplest formulations possible (with few ingredients).*

※ *Avoid products containing alcohol, which tends to dry out the skin.*

※ *Massage your skin daily with a suitable vegetable oil.*

~~~~

~~~~

MY FAVORITE PLANT OILS

※ *For drier skin: apricot, sweet almond, wheat germ, evening primrose, argan*

※ *For oily skin: jojoba, camellia, hazelnut, macadamia, melon*

※ *For sensitive skin: jojoba, calendula, raspberry, borage, prickly pear*

~~~~

THE PREGNANCY MASK

The chloasma or "pregnancy mask" is one inconvenience a pregnant woman may experience. It is characterized by brown spots that appear on the face. About 70 percent of women are affected by this hyperpigmentation of the skin. This phenomenon is the result of an increase in hormone levels that lead to a higher synthesis of melanin.

GOOD HABITS

❋ *Avoid sun exposure, which accentuates the spots.*

❋ *Use natural skin care products with mineral-based UV filters and without nanoparticles.*

❋ *Apply appropriate products, with plant extracts that have natural lightening properties.*

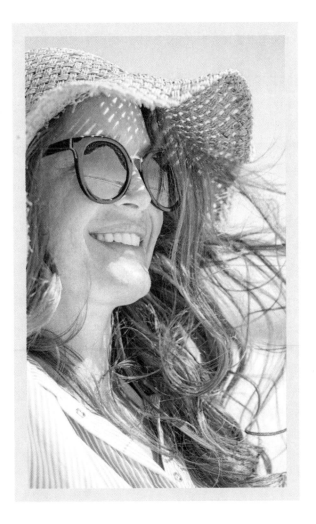

DELICATE CAMELLIA DAY CREAM

The combination of camellia oil, aloe vera gel, and lemon hydrosol makes this cream a treat for dull and tired complexions.

Preparation time: 20 min
Storage: 4 months
Materials: scale, bowl, pan, mini whisk, spatula
Packaging: 50 ml jar or pump bottle

INGREDIENTS

- 10 g camellia oil
- 5 g evening primrose oil
- 4 g vegetable emulsifying wax (Végémulse or Olivem 1000)
- 20 g aloe vera gel
- 10 g lemon hydrosol
- 2 drops natural vitamin E
- 6 drops Cosgard preservative

PREPARATION

Pour all the ingredients except the Cosgard into a heat-resistant bowl, then make a water bath: fill a saucepan with water, set over low heat, and place the bowl on top of the saucepan. Once the emulsifying wax is completely melted, remove the bowl from the water bath and start emulsifying with a whisk. When the cream is opaque and creamy, add the preservative and mix for a few moments using a spatula. Transfer the cream to its container.

DIRECTIONS FOR USE

Apply a few drops of cream to clean, dry skin, starting from the center of the face and working outward. Don't forget the neck and upper chest.

TIP

DURING PREGNANCY

To soothe cramps, for a few minutes massage the area of the foot in between where the bone of the big toe joins with the bone of the second toe. This acupuncture point allows the tendons and muscles to relax and relieves cramps.

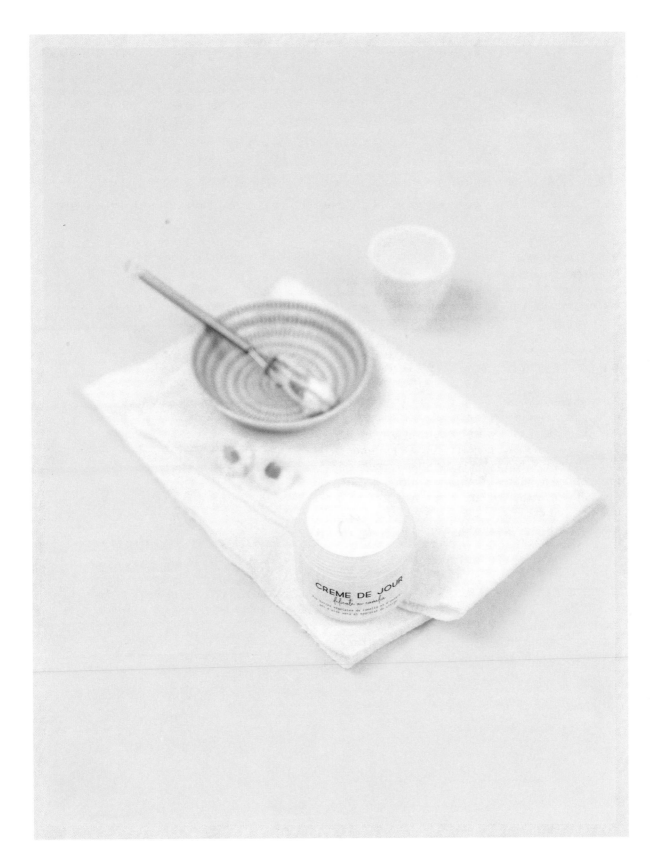

REGENERATING AVOCADO NIGHT CREAM

Rich in antioxidants and silica, this cream stimulates collagen synthesis to make the skin supple and elastic while restoring the hydrolipidic film.

Preparation time: 20 min
Storage: 4 months
Materials: scale, bowl, pan, mini whisk, spatula
Packaging: 50 ml jar or pump bottle

PREPARATION

Pour all the ingredients except the Cosgard into a heat-resistant bowl, then make a water bath: fill a saucepan with water, set over low heat, and place the bowl on top of the saucepan. Once the emulsifying wax is completely melted, remove the bowl from the water bath and start emulsifying with a whisk. When the cream is opaque and creamy, add the preservative and mix for a few moments using a spatula. Transfer the cream to its container.

DIRECTIONS FOR USE

Apply a few drops of cream to clean, dry skin, starting from the center of the face and working outward. Don't forget the neck and upper chest.

INGREDIENTS

- 10 g jojoba oil
- 5 g avocado oil
- 4 g vegetable emulsifying wax (Végémulse or Olivem 1000)
- 25 g bamboo hydrosol
- 5 g vegetable glycerin
- 2 drops natural vitamin E
- 6 drops Cosgard preservative

TIP

FOR GASTRIC ACIDITY

In the evening, allow 2 teaspoons of green clay powder to settle in a large glass of water. In the morning, drink this clay water on an empty stomach.

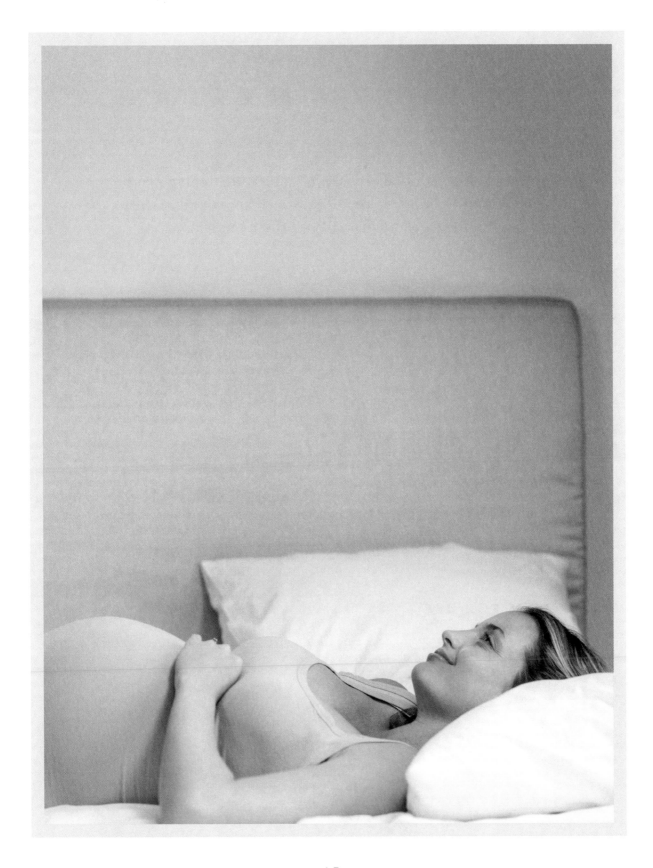

WHITE LILY RADIANT COMPLEXION CREAM

This cream is a powerhouse of natural lightening plant extracts. It lightens or removes brown spots and restores radiance and luminosity to the complexion.

Preparation time: 20 min
Storage: 4 months
Materials: scale, bowl, pan, mini whisk, spatula
Packaging: 50 ml jar or pump bottle

INGREDIENTS

- 15 g white lily macerated oil
- 4 g vegetable emulsifying wax (Végémulse or Olivem 1000)
- 20 g lemon hydrosol
- 5 g vegetable glycerin
- 2 drops natural vitamin E
- 15 drops active AHA (fruit acids)
- 6 drops Cosgard preservative

PREPARATION

Pour all the ingredients except the active AHA and Cosgard into a heat-resistant bowl, then make a water bath: fill a saucepan with water, set over low heat, and place the bowl on top of the saucepan. Once the emulsifying wax is completely melted, remove the bowl from the water bath and start emulsifying with a whisk. When the cream is opaque and creamy, add the active AHA followed by the preservative, then mix with a spatula for a few moments. Transfer the cream to its container.

DIRECTIONS FOR USE

Apply a few drops of cream to clean, dry skin, starting from the center of the face and working outward. Don't forget the neck and upper chest.

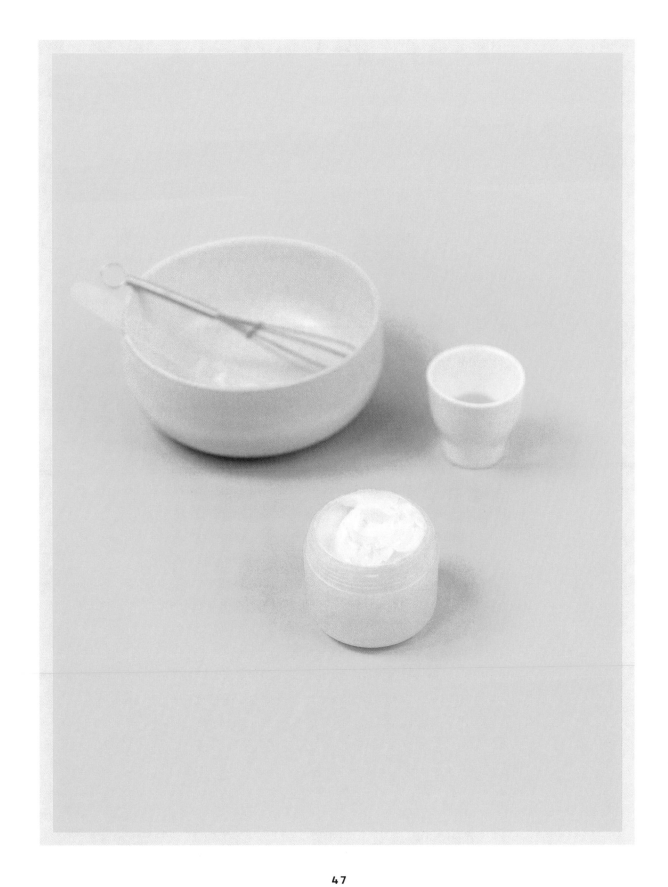

BRIGHTENING ACEROLA MASK

Acerola, a small Amazonian fruit also known as the "Barbados cherry," contains twenty to thirty times more vitamin C than an orange and is also rich in minerals. It naturally prevents the epithelial cells from producing the melanin that causes skin pigmentation.

Preparation time: 5 min
Storage: to be used immediately
Materials: bowl, wooden or porcelain spoon
Packaging: none

INGREDIENTS

- 2 tablespoons pink clay
- 2 tablespoons apricot oil
- 1/2 teaspoon acerola powder

PREPARATION

In a bowl, combine the clay and apricot oil, then add the acerola powder, stirring until the mixture is consistent. Never use metal utensils to prepare your clay-based masks.

DIRECTIONS FOR USE

Apply the mixture to the skin in a thick layer. Leave on for 15 minutes, then remove the mask with a damp cloth. Finish with a spray of floral water. Do not allow the clay to dry on the skin: if necessary, moisten it regularly during the application time by spraying a little floral or mineral water.

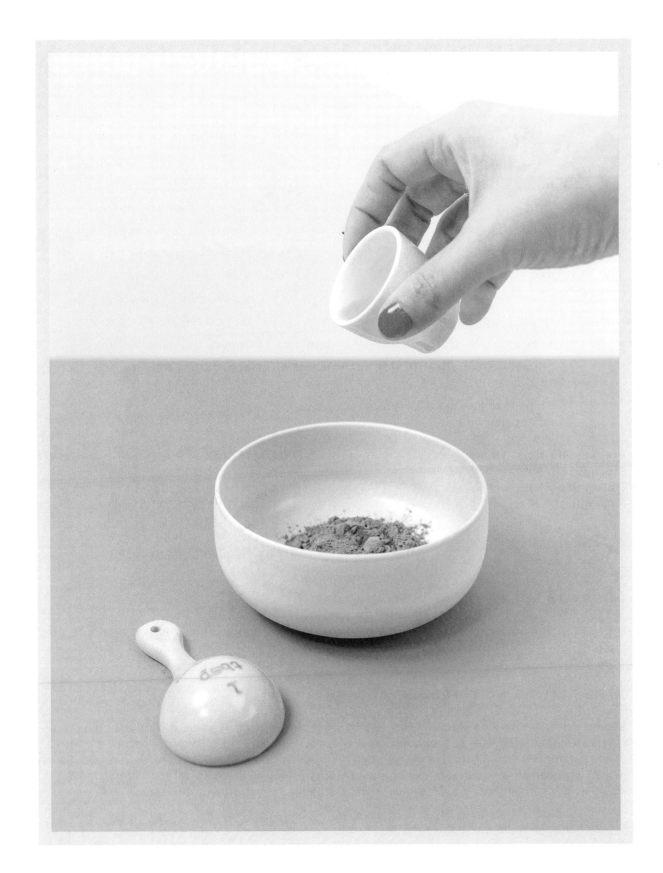

ANTI-ROSACEA SERUM

Because pregnancy hormones cause the small blood vessels in the skin to dilate, pregnant women frequently suffer from rosacea (in around one out of three cases). It disappears after the baby is born. In addition, small, blood-red dots (spider angioma) may appear on the face and décolletage or take the form of fine cobwebs (spider telangiectasia). These lesions are not serious and spontaneously regress after childbirth. Safflower oil, which is rich in vitamin K, promotes microcirculation in the skin and reduces the appearance of small vessels. Hemp oil is soothing and restorative; it restores softness and elasticity to the skin and restructures cell membranes. Tamanu oil helps to strengthen the skin and calm redness.

Preparation time: 10 min
Storage: 3 months
Materials: scale
Packaging: 100 ml pump bottle

INGREDIENTS

- 60 g witch hazel hydrosol
- 30 g Douglas fir hydrosol
- 2 g xanthan gum
- 8 g tamanu oil
- 20 drops Cosgard preservative

PREPARATION

Pour the ingredients into the bottle one by one. Close the bottle, then shake it gently to mix the oils.

DIRECTIONS FOR USE

Squeeze 3 or 4 drops of serum into the palm of your hand, then warm it up by rubbing your palms together. Massage in a circular motion on areas prone to rosacea (sides of the nose, cheeks, temples), on clean skin. Then apply your usual cream. To help the serum penetrate better, you can spray your skin generously with hydrosol or thermal water (without letting it dry) just prior to application. This way, it will not leave an oily film on the skin.

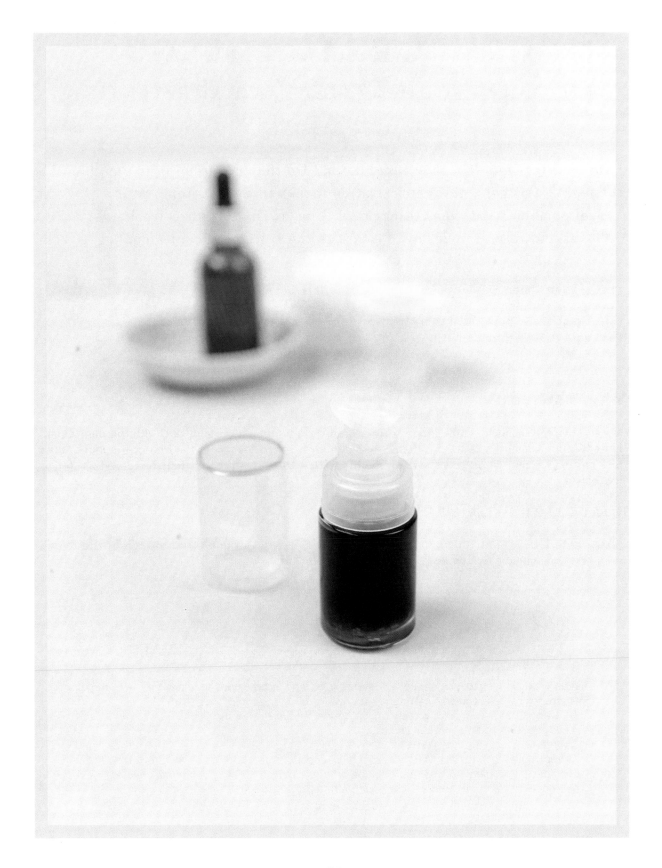

GEL FOR LIGHT LEGS
TREATMENT FOR HEAVY LEGS, WATER RETENTION

~~~

Do your legs feel like they weigh a ton? Do they cramp up in the middle of the night? This gel activates circulation thanks to the vasotonic action of witch hazel combined with the freshness of Douglas fir. This ultra-fresh gel gently relieves and relaxes your legs. Place it in the refrigerator for a cooling effect.

Preparation time: 10 min
Storage: 3 months
Materials: scale, bowl, mini whisk
Packaging: 100 ml pump bottle

INGREDIENTS

60 g witch hazel hydrosol
30 g Douglas fir hydrosol
2 g xanthan gum
8 g tamanu oil
20 drops Cosgard preservative

PREPARATION

Mix the two hydrosols in a bowl, then sprinkle in the xanthan gum while mixing with the mini whisk. Let stand for 5 minutes so the xanthan gum completely rehydrates. Add the rest of the ingredients one by one, mixing vigorously between each addition to obtain a consistent texture. Transfer to the bottle.

DIRECTIONS FOR USE

Shake before use. Apply this gel starting at the ankles and working up to the top of the thighs with long massaging movements to activate circulation.

GOOD HABITS

* *When you are lying down, remember to raise your legs a few inches to improve blood circulation.*
* *Massage yourself regularly, moving up from your feet to the top of your thighs.*
* *Shower your legs with cold water, working up toward the tops of the thighs.*
* *Avoid exposing your legs to the sun.*
* *Limit the amount of salt in your diet.*
* *Certain plants taken in the form of herbal teas, capsules, or ampoules can improve blood circulation, including red vine (protects the arteries, vasoconstrictor) and horse chestnut (increases capillary resistance). Ask your pharmacist for advice.*

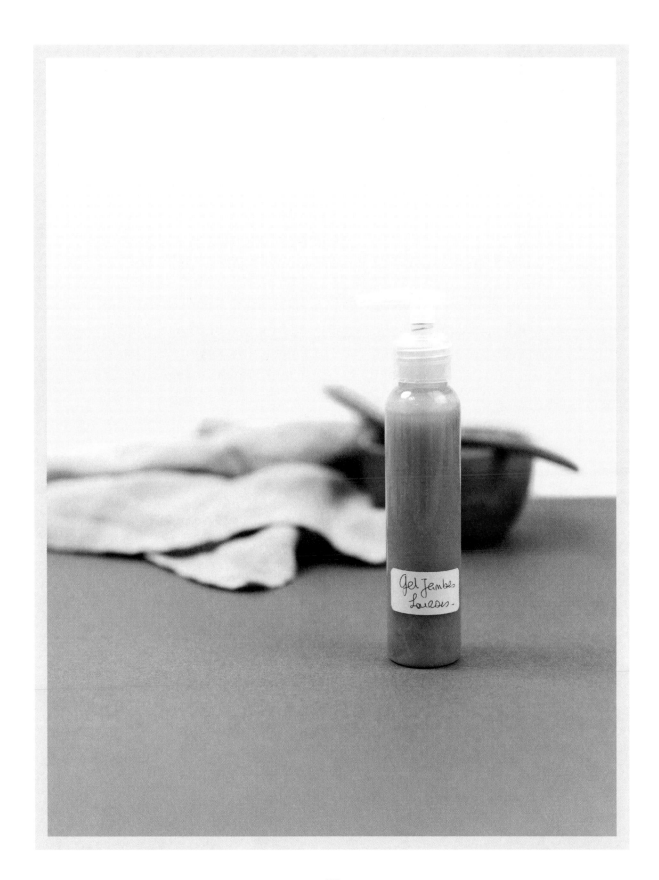

ANTI-STRETCH MARK TREATMENTS

~~~~~~~~

Stretch marks are simply unfair! Some people conscientiously apply cream and oil all throughout their pregnancy but still suffer from these invasive stripes, while others who have taken no preventative measures don't get a single one

Though genetics do play a part, anti-stretch mark creams and oils can help keep your skin supple and even fade those unsightly marks. So be sure to take care of your breasts, your thighs, in and of course your belly by massaging them in regularly.

~~~~~~~~

GOOD HABITS

Essential fatty acids as well as vitamins from the B, C, and E groups keep the skin supple and smooth while boosting the production of collagen. Consider taking evening primrose oil and wheat germ oil, which provide the fatty acids necessary to prevent stretch marks and strengthen the skin's structure. You can find these plant oils in capsule form in pharmacies and health food stores.

~~~~~~~~

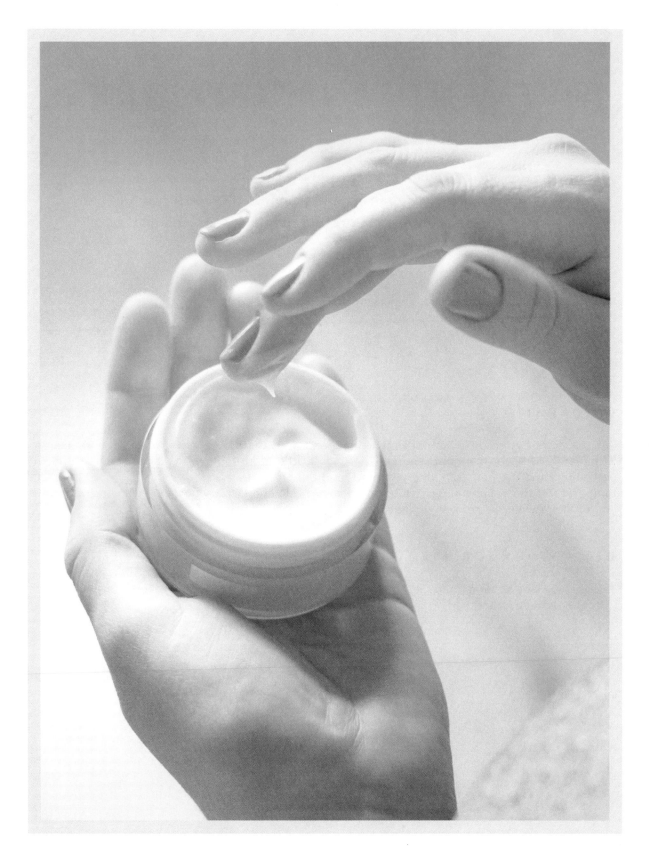

WHIPPED BALM TO PREVENT STRETCH MARKS

~~~~~~~~

Avocado and macadamia oils are known to be extremely softening and regenerating. Repairing and calming, they work wonders on skin prone to discomfort and help fight stretch marks.

Preparation time: 20 min
Storage: 12 months
Materials: scale, bowl, pan, mini whisk
Packaging: 100 ml glass jar

INGREDIENTS

- 30 g cocoa butter
- 30 g shea butter
- 20 g macadamia oil
- 20 g avocado oil
- 5 drops natural vitamin E

PREPARATION

Put the plant butters in a heat-resistant bowl and melt them in a water bath: fill a saucepan with water, set over low heat, and set the bowl in the pan. Remove the bowl from the water bath, then add the plant oils and vitamin E and stir for a few seconds. Allow to cool to room temperature; the balm will become translucent. At this point, mix vigorously with a whisk until you obtain a whipped texture. Transfer to the jar.

DIRECTIONS FOR USE

Take a large dab of balm, then massage the affected areas in circular movements until the balm is completely absorbed.

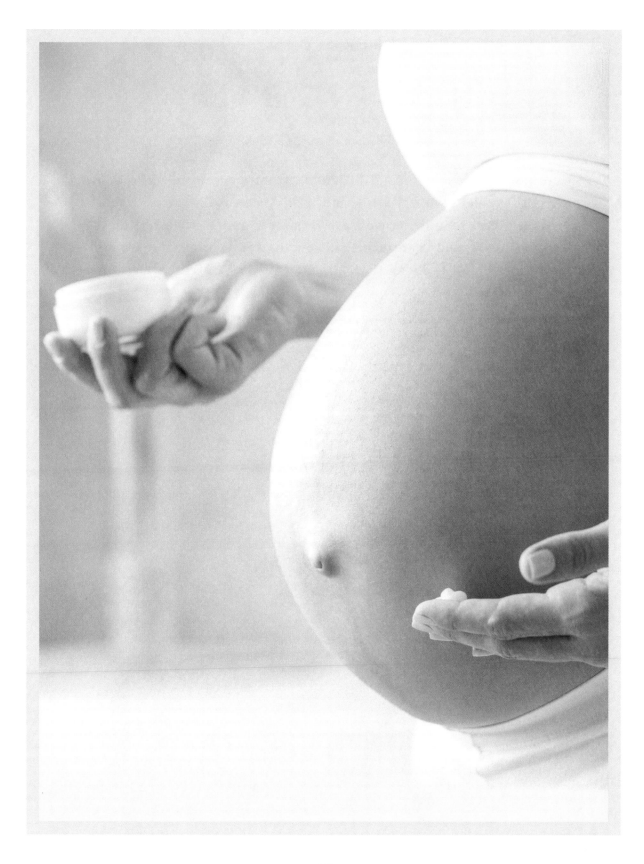

ANTI-STRETCH MARK HEALING BALM

~~~~~~~~

Soothing and restructuring, St. John's wort macerated oil is known to fight against skin irritation and itching caused by stretch marks. Rich in carotenoids as well as vitamins E and K, rose hip oil is regenerative and restorative; it accelerates healing, boosts cell renewal, and reduces the redness caused by stretch marks.

Preparation time: 20 min
Storage: 9 months
Materials: scale, bowl, pan, mini whisk
Packaging: 100 ml glass jar

INGREDIENTS

30 g cocoa butter
30 g shea butter
20 g St. John's wort macerated oil
20 g rose hip oil
5 drops natural vitamin E

PREPARATION

Put the plant butters in a heat-resistant bowl and melt them in a water bath: fill a saucepan with water, set over low heat, and place the bowl in the pan. Remove the bowl from the water bath, then add the plant oils and and vitamin E and stir for a few seconds. Allow to cool to room temperature; the balm will become translucent. At this point, mix vigorously with a whisk until you obtain a whipped texture. Transfer to the jar.

DIRECTIONS FOR USE

Take a large dab of balm, then massage the areas where there are stretch marks, using circular movements until the balm is completely absorbed.

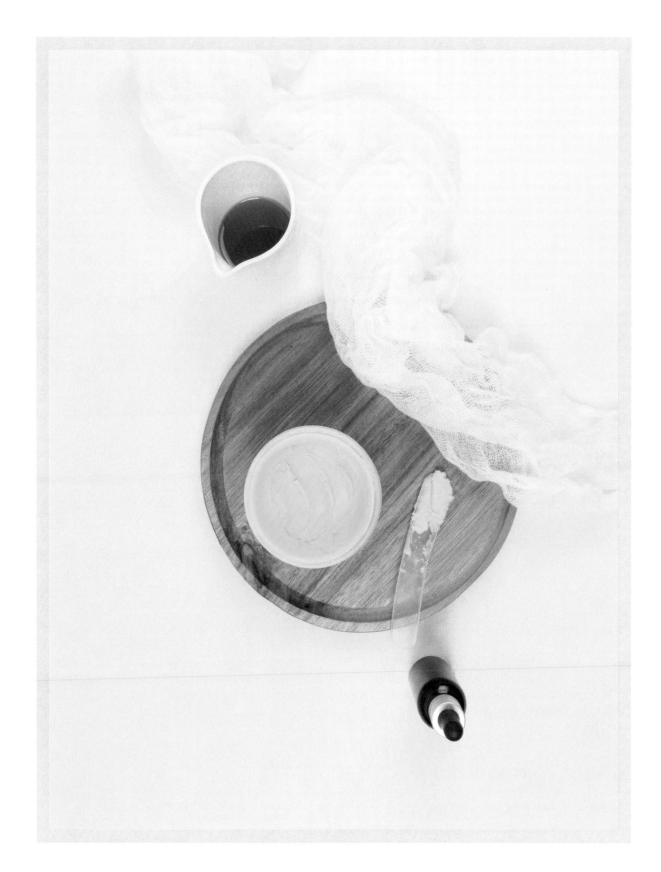

CREAM DEODORANT WITH COLLOIDAL SILVER

~~~~~~~~~

Commercially available deodorants are so saturated with questionable ingredients that there's no question you should avoid them while pregnant. There are other attractive solutions for combating perspiration and bad odors. Absorbent powders such as clay and certain starches absorb moisture while allowing toxins to escape naturally, and certain natural agents help to combat odors. Colloidal silver acts naturally against the bacteria that causes bad odors and leaves a pleasant sensation of freshness on the skin. Magnesium oxide is a natural antibacterial agent, while white clay and arrowroot are two powders that absorb moisture.

Preparation time: 15 min
Storage: 12 months
Materials: scale, bowl, pan, mini whisk
Packaging: 50 ml stick bottle

INGREDIENTS

10 g colloidal silver (20 ppm or more[4])
10 g arrowroot
5 g magnesium oxide powder
   (available in pharmacies)
5 g white clay
15 g shea butter
5 g candelilla wax

PREPARATION

In a bowl, mix the colloidal silver with the arrowroot, magnesium oxide, and clay. Add the rest of the ingredients and melt in a water bath: fill a saucepan with water, set over low heat, and place the bowl on top of the saucepan. Remove the bowl from the pan and whisk vigorously until the mixture becomes smooth. Transfer to the stick bottle and leave in the refrigerator for 30 minutes.

DIRECTIONS FOR USE

Apply deodorant to the armpits.

~~~~~~~~~

4   Dosed at 20 mg per liter. Available in health food stores.

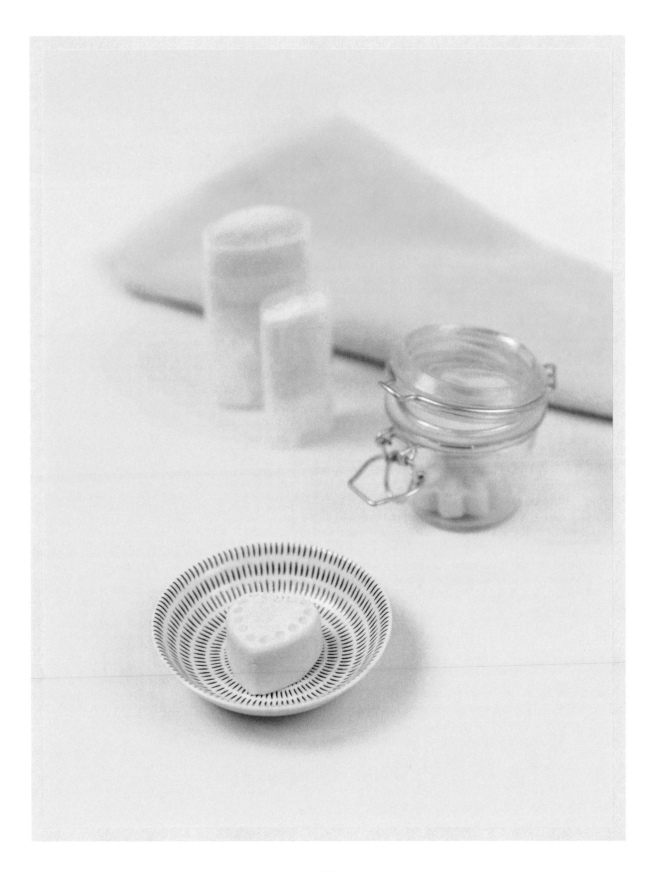

AROMATIC BALM
FOR BACK PAIN AND SCIATICA

During pregnancy, the baby grows in the uterus and the pelvis expands. As it expands, it can sometimes press on the nerve, causing pain and sometimes even immobilization.

Precautions: do not use in first trimester of pregnancy.
Preparation time: 15 min
Storage: 12 months
Materials: scale, bowl, pan, spatula
Packaging: 10 ml jar

INGREDIENTS

- 3 g beeswax
- 3 g shea butter
- 4 g arnica macerated oil
- 10 drops true lavender essential oil (Lavandula angustifolia)

PREPARATION

Combine the beeswax, shea butter, and arnica oil in a heat-resistant bowl and melt them in a water bath: fill a saucepan with water, set over low heat, and place the bowl on top of the saucepan. Remove from heat and stir until the mixture becomes translucent, then add the essential oil and mix quickly. Transfer to the jar before it sets.

DIRECTIONS FOR USE

Scoop out some of the balm and let it melt on your fingers. Massage onto the sensitive area 2 to 3 times a day for a maximum of 5 days.

TIP

LOWER-BACK STRETCH

Lie on your back, grab your knees, and bring your chin toward your neck. While exhaling, spread your knees apart and try to pull them up under your arms by bending your elbows outward and upward. Repeat several times.

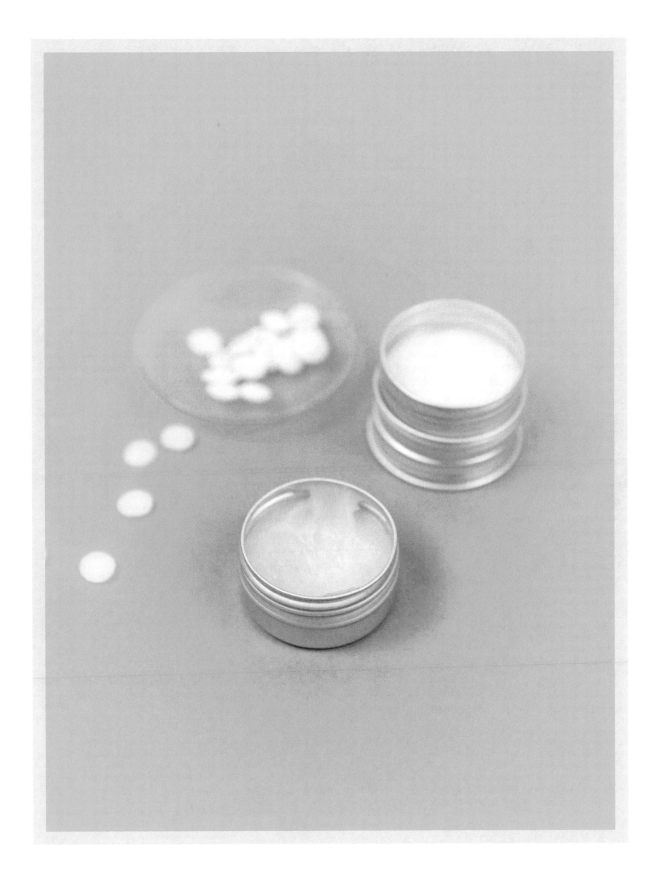

ANTI-NAUSEA BALM

~~~

Lemon essence has mild anti-nausea properties and is a digestive tonic. It contains terpenes, which help with gastric mobility and improve digestion. Inhaling it via the respiratory tract is gentle and less intrusive than taking it orally.

GOOD HABITS

Drink a glass of fresh lemon juice in the morning when you wake up. A hepatic regenerator and antiseptic, lemon promotes digestive function. Spread out your meals. A few slices of banana can stop nausea. Rich in vitamin B6, banana is also extremely valuable in the development of your future baby's nervous system.

Precautions: photosensitizing essential oil; avoid sun exposure for 8 hours following application.
Preparation time: 15 min
Storage: 12 months
Materials: scale, bowl, pan, spatula
Packaging: 10 ml jar

INGREDIENTS

3 g beeswax
3 g shea butter
4 g sweet almond oil
10 drops lemon essence

PREPARATION

Combine the beeswax, shea butter, and sweet almond oil in a heat-resistant bowl and melt them in a water bath: fill a saucepan with water, set over low heat, and place the bowl on top of the saucepan. Remove from the heat and stir until the mixture becomes translucent, then add the lemon essence and stir quickly. Transfer to the jar before it sets.

DIRECTIONS FOR USE

Scoop out some of the balm and let it melt on your fingers. Apply by massaging to the insides of the wrists in a circular motion. Breathe in the vapors from the mixture.

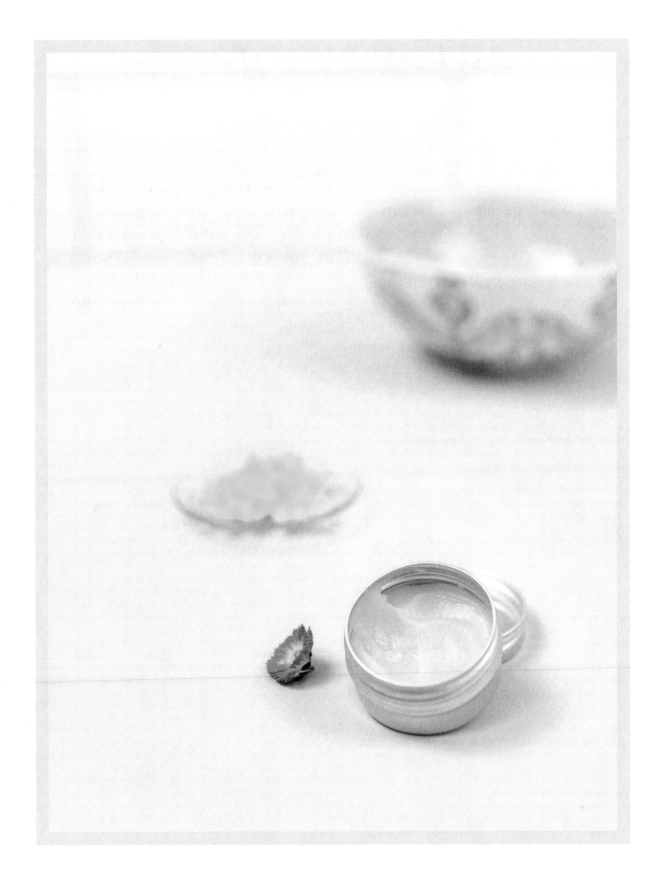

ANTI-HEARTBURN AROMATIC BALM

Heartburn occurs during pregnancy for two main reasons. First, to relax progesterone causes the muscles in the digestive system to relax; digestion is not only slower, but the valve that connects the stomach to the esophagus may be sluggish and allow gastric juices to escape. As the pregnancy progresses and the fetus grows, the uterus presses on the stomach, causing it to rise upward. Traditionally, Roman chamomile is used to improve digestive comfort and facilitate sleep. Its essential oil has powerful antispasmodic properties, ideal for fighting heartburn even during pregnancy.

Precautions: photosensitizing essential oil; avoid sun exposure for 8 hours following application. Do not use in first trimester of pregnancy.
Preparation time: 15 min
Storage: 12 months
Materials: scale, bowl, pan, spatula
Packaging: 10 ml jar

INGREDIENTS

- 3 g beeswax
- 3 g shea butter
- 4 g sweet almond oil
- 5 drops Roman chamomile essential oil (Chamaemelum nobile)
- 5 drops mandarin orange essence (Citrus reticulata)

PREPARATION

Combine the beeswax, shea butter, and sweet almond oil in a heat-resistant bowl and melt them in a water bath: fill a saucepan with water, set over low heat, and place the bowl on top of the saucepan. Remove from the heat and stir until the mixture becomes translucent, then add the essential oils and mix quickly. Transfer to the jar before it sets. Let cool for 12 hours.

DIRECTIONS FOR USE

Scoop out some of the balm and let it melt on your fingers. Massage onto the solar plexus in circular motions, 2 to 3 times a day.

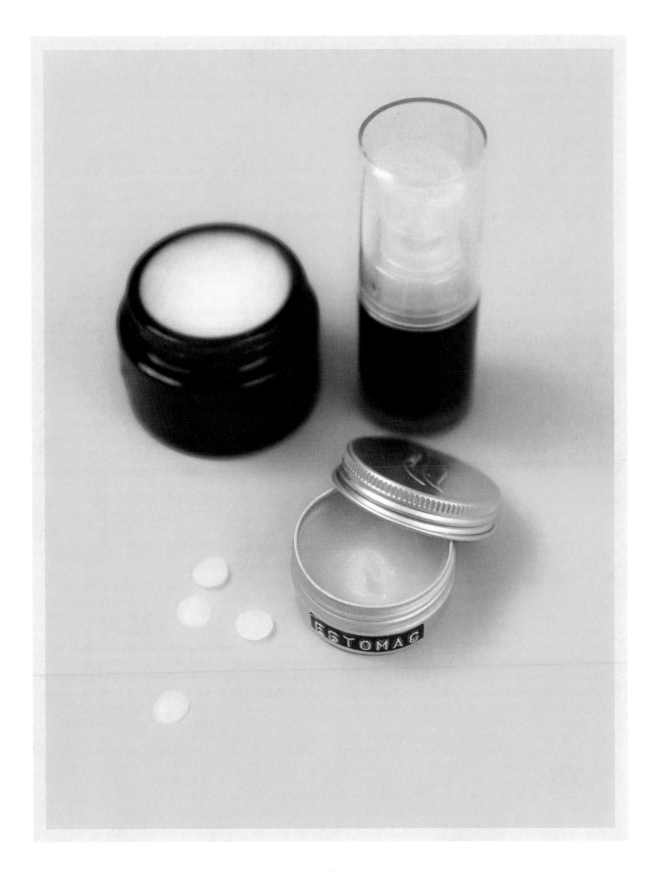

AFTER CHILDBIRTH

By Hélène Boyé, naturalist midwife

~~~~~~~~~~

After the birth comes the time for new habits and a new lifestyle.
It's a time to take care of your baby and integrate your child into the
family, but without forgetting to take care of yourself and your body.
It's also a time for physical recovery and emotional adjustment.

According to traditional Chinese medicine, the pregnant woman and the young mother should enjoy themselves, look at beautiful things, listen to beautiful music, and breathe in pleasant smells. In order to properly give and provide, the mother herself needs to be well.

Be attentive to your breastfeeding. Get support and advice from professionals who will be up on the latest findings and know how to talk to you about you and your baby.

Breastfeeding is a natural process, but that doesn't mean that it's easy in practice. Sometimes new mothers need support to help them make this connection to the baby.

Don't forget that physical, skin-to-skin contact with baby promotes the production of milk—so there's no limit to how much you can cuddle your baby! Newborns don't have any habits or throw tantrums, so it's a good idea to practice babywearing—that way, you're in physical contact as often as possible. Babywearing creates a feeling of protection and security. You can adapt your system so it makes your daily activities easier.

It's important to keep your baby in the right physiological position: the baby should be carried vertically, with the knees higher than the pelvis, and carried relatively high, with the head in line with the spine.

Take care of yourself by drinking plenty of water or herbal tea. The body and tissues need to be hydrated, especially while breastfeeding. Fennel seed, lemon balm, and anise herbal tea promote milk production and digestive comfort for the baby.

The body needs to be replenished with energy. Nutritious food and acupuncture, for example, will help you get back into shape quickly, especially if you are losing a lot of sleep while keeping watch over your baby at night.

Keep having what you want, but without overdoing it. Drink a lot of fluids, such as fresh fruit juices, in between meals. Opt for sweet flavors like beet, fennel, sweet potato, and carrot. Eggplant is subtle and fresh, nourishes the skin, and stimulates physical strength. It is particularly recommended during breastfeeding. Season your salads or cooked vegetables with cold-pressed plant oils such as sunflower, olive, and rapeseed.

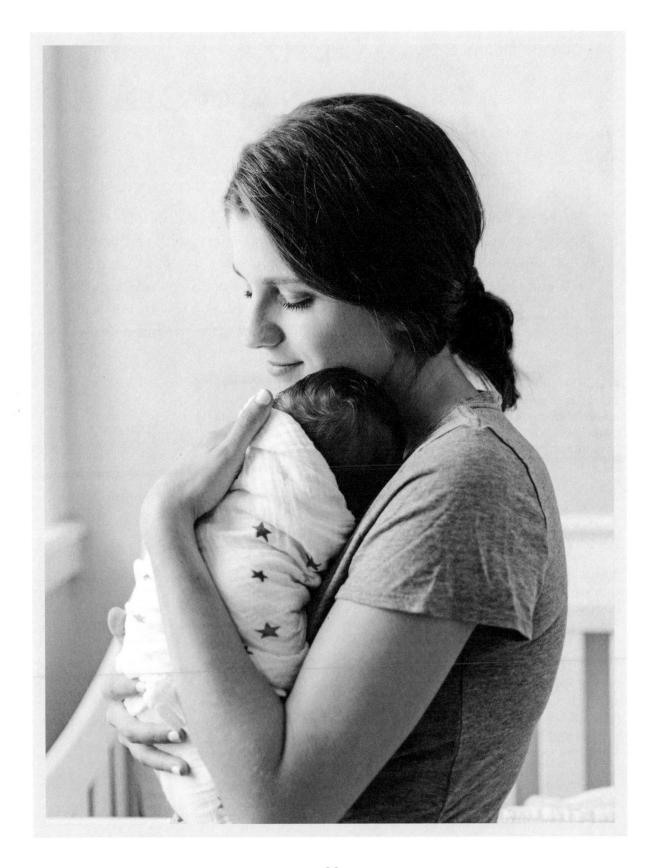

SOLID OATMEAL SHAMPOO
WITH GROWTH ACTIVATOR

Some women get beautiful, shiny, strong hair thanks to the effects of hormones; others find that their hair becomes short, dull, and brittle. A few months after giving birth, the hair often loses its volume and falls out, sometimes by the handful. Don't worry, this is completely natural! Castor and avocado oils are known to activate blood flow to the scalp to boost hair growth, while oatmeal softens sensitive, irritated scalps.

Preparation time: 20 min
Storage: 9 months
Materials: scale, bowl, pan, spatula, silicone mold (with 100 g capacity)
Packaging: none

INGREDIENTS

- 60 g SCI surfactant
- 10 g colloidal oat powder
- 10 g castor oil
- 10 g avocado oil
- 5 g vegetable glycerin
- 5 g spring water (or nettle hydrosol)

PREPARATION

Pour all the ingredients into a heat-resistant bowl and melt them in a water bath: fill a saucepan with water, set over low heat, and place the bowl on top of the saucepan. Once the paste is thick but uniform, remove from the heat, mix gently, and pour the mixture into a silicone mold. Press firmly. Let it harden overnight at room temperature, then remove from the mold. Leave the shampoo to air-dry for 3 days before using it for the first time.

DIRECTIONS FOR USE

Wet your hair thoroughly, then rub the solid shampoo on your scalp for several seconds until you get a dense lather. Massage your scalp with your fingertips to distribute the product evenly. Rinse thoroughly.

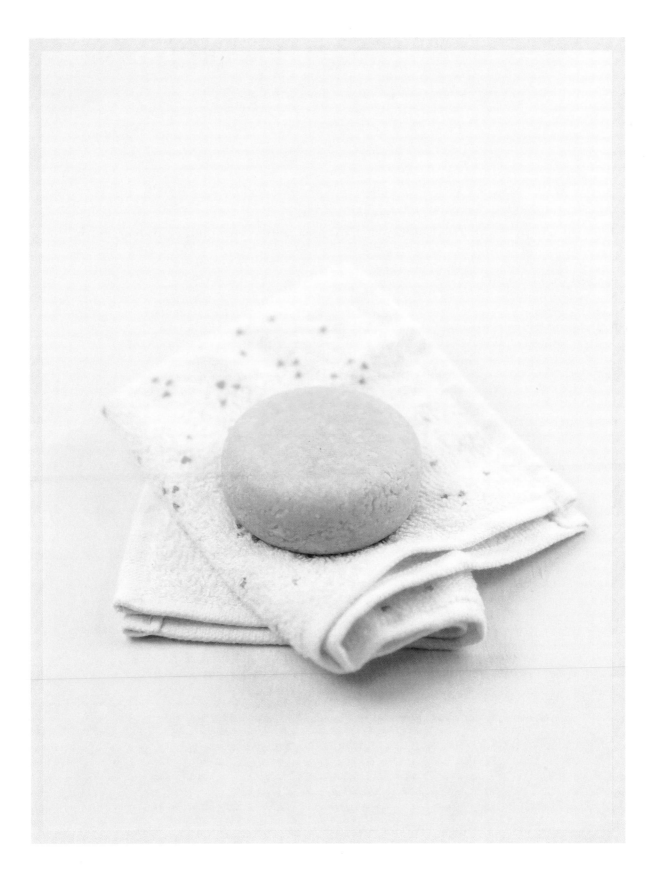

HAIR SERUM TO PREVENT HAIR LOSS

The synergy of natural active ingredients makes this serum an invigorating treatment specially designed to compensate for scalp imbalances and to slow down hair loss while stimulating hair growth.

Preparation time: 10 min
Storage: 4 months
Material: scale
Packaging: 100 ml spray bottle

INGREDIENTS

- 48 g nettle hydrosol (or nettle infusion)
- 1 g castor oil
- 1 g (or 25 drops) panthenol (provitamin B5)
- 6 drops Cosgard preservative

PREPARATION

Pour the ingredients one by one into the bottle, close it, and shake vigorously.

DIRECTIONS FOR USE

Shake vigorously before use. After shampooing, spray on hair while it is still damp. Rub your scalp for a few minutes. Do not rinse.

MY FAVORITE OILS

- *Oily hair: sesame, jojoba, hazelnut*
- *Dry hair: macadamia, baobab, argan, olive, coconut*
- *Hair loss: avocado, castor oil, pumpkin seed, mustard (to be diluted at 50 percent)*

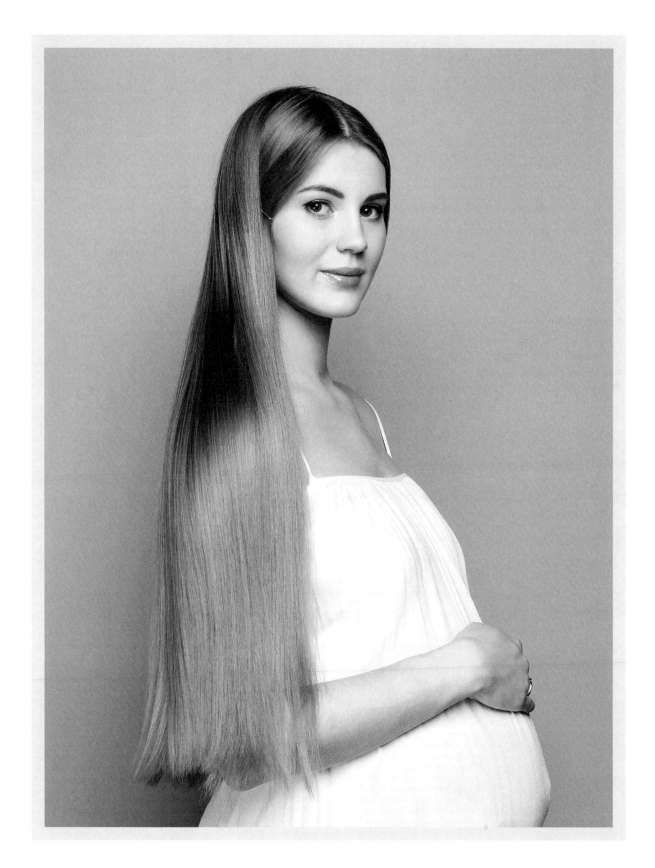

ANTI-FATIGUE EYE SERUM

~~~~~~~

Tamanu oil is an anti-inflammatory and a stimulant that activates circulation in the vessels to reduce the dark color of circles under the eyes, while cucumber oil reduces puffiness. Argan and avocado oils act as antiaging agents without causing the eyes to swell.

Preparation time: 5 min
Storage: 12 months
Material: scale
Packaging: 10 ml roll-on bottle

INGREDIENTS

❋ 3 g argan oil
❋ 3 g avocado oil
❋ 2 g cucumber oil
❋ 2 g tamanu oil

PREPARATION

Pour the ingredients one by one into the bottle, close it, then shake it gently until the oils are well-blended.

DIRECTIONS FOR USE

On clean skin, glide the roll-on from the inside to the outside of the eyes. Then tap your skin with your fingertips to help the serum absorb.

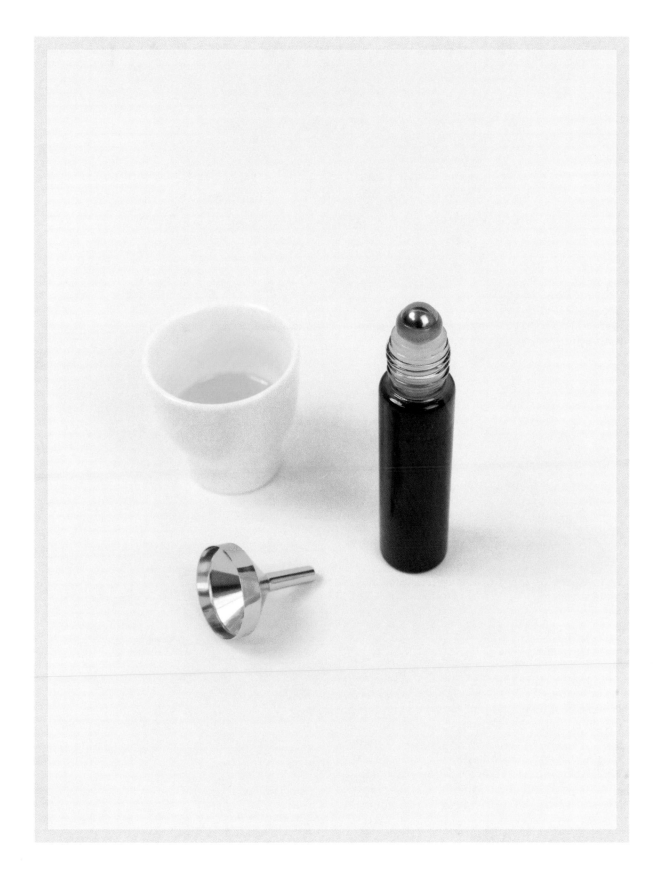

FIRMING BODY CREAM
WITH GRAPEFRUIT

~~~~~~~

After 9 months of pregnancy, the skin tissues are weakened and slack. A daily massage using a firming treatment that is both effective and breastfeeding-compatible is ideal.

Preparation time: 20 min
Storage: 9 months
Materials: scale, bowl, pan, mini whisk, spatula
Packaging: 100 ml glass jar

INGREDIENTS

- 8 g shea butter
- 8 g avocado oil
- 8 g macadamia oil
- 8 g rose hip oil
- 8 g vegetable emulsifying wax (Végémulse or Olivem 1000)
- 55 g spring water
- 5 g vegetable glycerin
- 5 drops natural vitamin E
- 30 drops grapefruit essential oil
- 16 drops Cosgard preservative

PREPARATION

Pour all the ingredients except the essential oil and the Cosgard into a heat-resistant bowl, then make a water bath: fill a saucepan with water, set over low heat, and place the bowl on top of the saucepan. As soon as the emulsifying wax is completely melted, remove the bowl from the water bath and start emulsifying with a whisk. When the cream becomes opaque and creamy, add the essential oil and then the preservative. Mix with a spatula for a few seconds. Pour the cream into the jar.

DIRECTIONS FOR USE

Apply generously to areas to be firmed like the stomach, buttocks, and thighs.

~~~~~~~

MY FAVORITE OILS

- *Anti-stretch marks: sesame, avocado, jojoba, sweet almond, argan, shea butter*

- *Firming and anti-cellulite: andiroba, babassu, borage, rose hip, cocoa butter, mango butter*

- *To combat crocodile skin: olive, macadamia, wheat germ, apricot, shea butter*

~~~~~~~

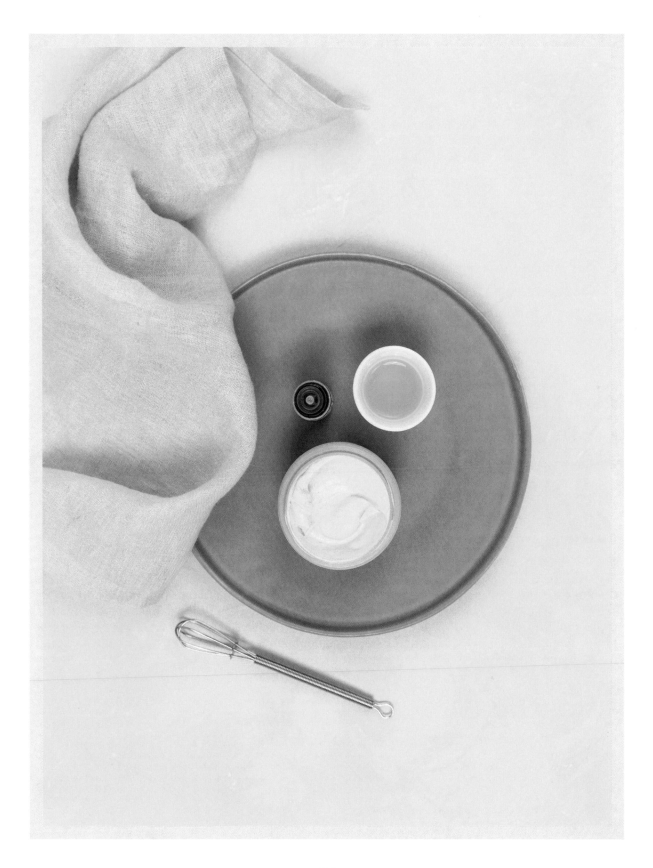

OINTMENT TO PROTECT AGAINST CRACKED SKIN WHILE BREASTFEEDING

This ointment is ideal for taking care of your breasts while breastfeeding. Massaging your breasts while applying this type of ointment helps prevent the appearance of cracks and improves conditions for breastfeeding.

Preparation time: 20 min
Storage: 12 months
Materials: scale, bowl, pan, mini whisk
Packaging: 50 ml jar

INGREDIENTS

✳ 10 g plant-based lanolin substitute
✳ 10 g shea butter
✳ 10 g St. John's wort macerated oil (or sweet almond oil)
✳ 3 g vegetable glycerin
✳ 2 drops natural vitamin E

PREPARATION

Combine all the ingredients in a heat-resistant bowl, then melt them in a water bath: fill a saucepan with water, set over low heat, and place the bowl on top of the saucepan. Remove the bowl from the water bath and whisk the mixture vigorously. Place the bowl in the refrigerator for 10 minutes, then stir again vigorously for about 2 minutes. Transfer to the jar. Let stand for 12 hours.

DIRECTIONS FOR USE

After breastfeeding, apply a small amount of ointment to the nipples and massage gently.

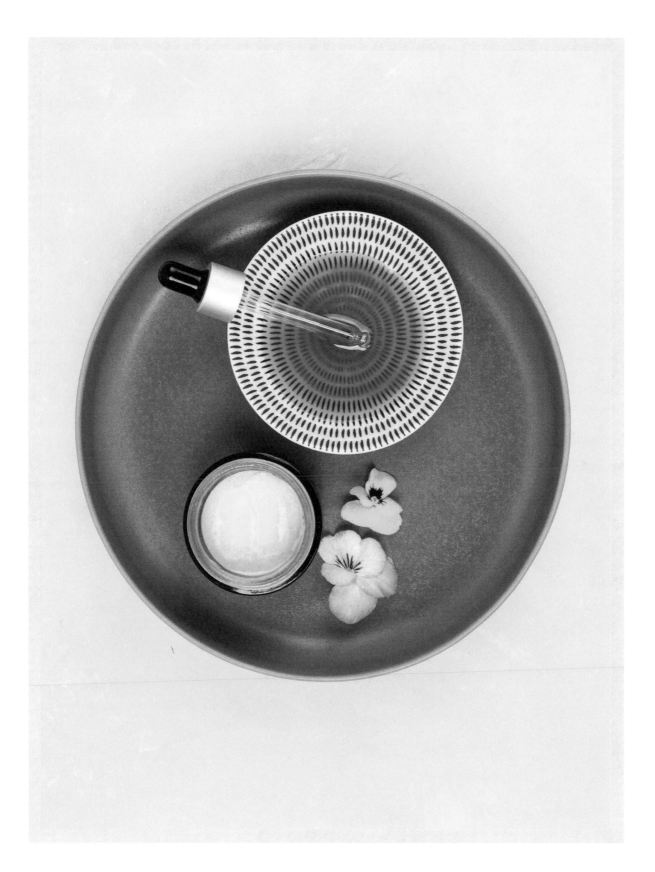

"PUSH-UP" DAISY FLUID

~~~~~~~~

Rich in active tensing agents, this fluid for the chest gives shape to the bust and strengthens the tissues. The firming qualities of the daisy (Bellis) are accentuated by the reshaping and tightening effects of aloe vera. Rich in vitamin C and trace elements, acerola helps to restore the skin's elasticity and firmness. This fluid and matte gel-cream absorbs quickly and leaves the skin soft.

Preparation time: 10 min
Storage: 4 months
Materials: scale, bowl, mini whisk
Packaging: 100 ml pump bottle

INGREDIENTS

- 8 g vegetable glycerin
- 1 g acerola powder (optional)
- 60 g aloe vera gel
- 30 g daisy macerated oil (Bellis)
- 16 drops Cosgard preservative
- 2 drops natural vitamin E

PREPARATION

In a bowl, mix the glycerin and acerola, then add the aloe vera gel. Gradually incorporate the daisy macerated oil while stirring with a whisk. Add the rest of the ingredients and stir again for 2 minutes. Transfer to the bottle.

DIRECTIONS FOR USE

Shake vigorously before use. Apply daily by massaging from the base of the breasts to the chin, paying particular attention to the upper part of the chest.

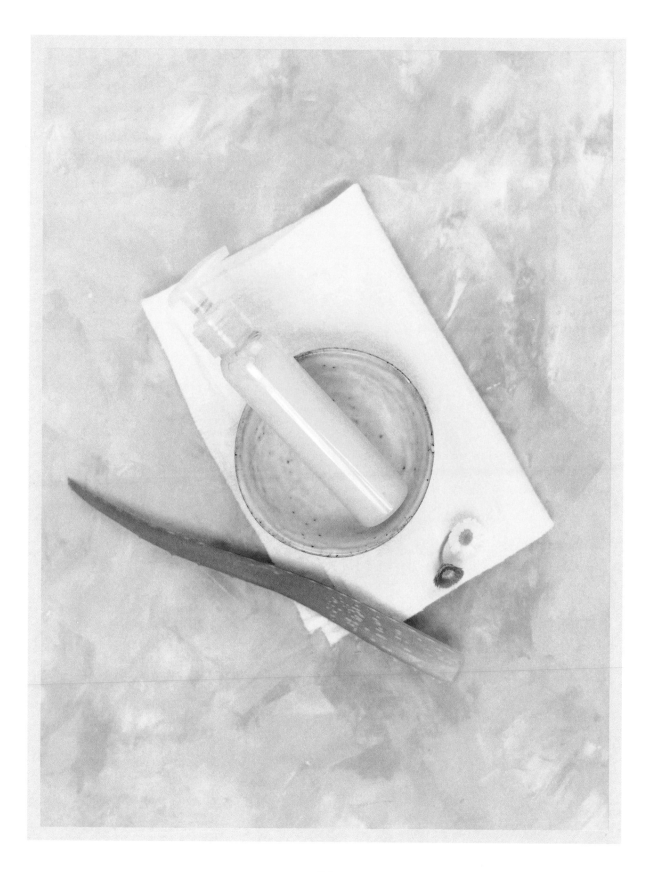

INTIMATE CLEANSING GEL

As the baby is being born, there may be small ruptures to your skin. The obstetrician might perform an episiotomy (an incision that makes it easier for the baby to pass through), which can cause pain or tingling. With the right bodywork and products, everything will return to normal within a few days.

Preparation time: 10 min
Storage: 4 months
Materials: scale, bowl, spatula
Packaging: 100 ml pump bottle

INGREDIENTS

- 35 g spring water
- 30 g vegetable glycerin
- 15 g aloe vera gel
- 15 g lauryl glucoside (base consistency)
- 5 g coco glucoside (douceur de coco)
- 20 drops Cosgard preservative

PREPARATION

Pour the ingredients one by one into a bowl, mixing gently with a spatula between each addition. Transfer to the bottle.

DIRECTIONS FOR USE

Use in the shower for intimate cleansing.

EXPRESS RECIPE
SOOTHING POULTICE

- Mix 1 tablespoon of powdered green clay and 1 tablespoon of spring water (or hydrosol) in order to obtain a consistent paste, then apply it in a thick layer to the area to be treated.

- Leave the mixture on for 10 minutes, then rinse.

GOOD HABITS

- Intimate cleansing should be performed daily and with a product with an adapted pH.

- In case of episiotomy, a scar treatment oil can be applied to the scar.

- Opt for organic cotton underwear that lets the skin breathe.

- Do not use tampons during this time.

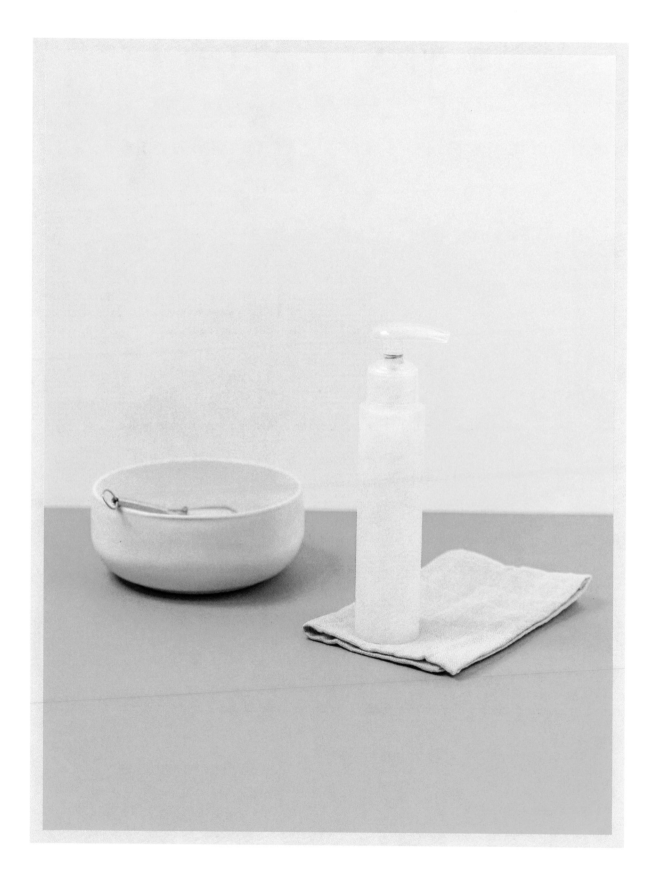

ULTRA-HEALING MEDICINAL OIL

FOR EPISIOTOMIES AND CAESAREAN SECTIONS

Preparation time: 5 min
Storage: 12 months
Material: scale
Packaging: 30 ml tinted glass bottle

INGREDIENTS

- 10 g rose hip oil
- 10 g arnica macerated oil
- 10 g St. John's wort macerated oil
- 22 drops Italian helichrysum essential oil (Helichrysum italicum)

PREPARATION

Pour all the ingredients into the bottle and shake for a few seconds to mix well.

DIRECTIONS FOR USE

Use 2 to 3 drops of this oil to perform a circular massage on the area of the episiotomy or caesarean section scar 2 to 4 times a day. Cover your belly when you are breastfeeding to keep the baby from coming into contact with the essential oils.

TIP

Consider an acupuncture session to promote blood microcirculation, which helps in the healing of wounds.

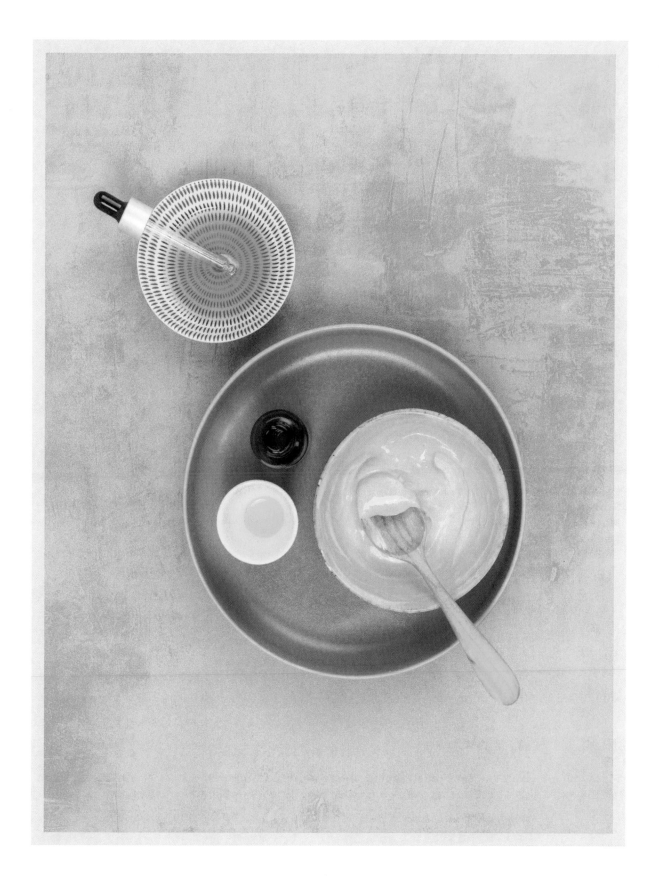

BABY BLUES AND POSTPARTUM DEPRESSION MASSAGE OIL

The baby blues is a short-lived slump and is milder than what is known as postpartum depression, which develops and worsens over time. Crying for no reason, being sad, and feeling overwhelmed or worthless are among the main symptoms. Hormonal changes, lack of family and social support, and fatigue can contribute to postpartum depression. The risk increases if the mother has previously suffered from depression. Here is a recipe that may help you, though it should not be used as a substitute for medical advice. In all cases, don't hesitate to talk about it with your doctor.

Preparation time: 10 min
Storage: 12 months
Material: scale
Packaging: 10 ml tinted glass bottle with dropper or pipette cap

INGREDIENTS

- 8 g hazelnut (or jojoba) oil
- 10 drops Roman chamomile essential oil (Chamaemelum nobile)
- 10 drops shell marjoram essential oils
- 10 drops small grain bitter orange essential oil (Citrus aurantium ssp. aurantium)

PREPARATION

Pour the ingredients one by one into the bottle. Close it, then shake it gently to mix the oils well. Wait 48 hours before use so that the active ingredients can synergize and intensify.

DIRECTIONS FOR USE

Massage immediately after breastfeeding. Apply 4 drops of oil on the solar plexus and 2 drops on the inner side of each wrist. Repeat applications twice a day until symptoms improve.

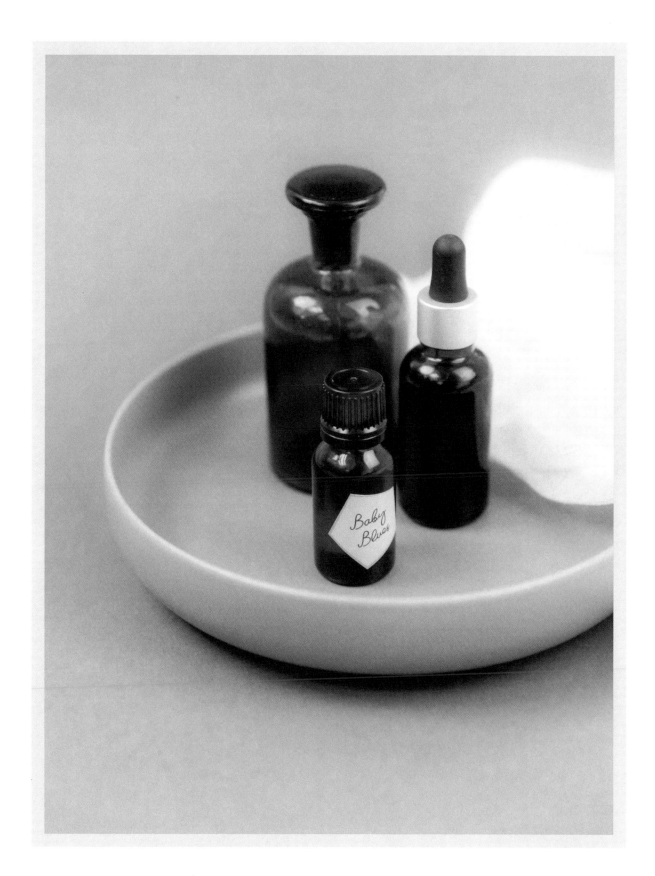

BABY BLUES ROOM FRAGRANCE

~~~~~~~~

Preparation time: 10 min
Storage: 6 months
Material: scale
Packaging: 50 ml spray bottle

INGREDIENTS

- 35 g 70 percent alcohol
- 15 g spring water
- 10 drops bergamot essential oil (Citrus aurantium bergamia)
- 10 drops geranium bourbon essential oil (Pelargonium asperum)
- 10 drops lemon litsea essential oil

PREPARATION

Pour the 70 percent alcohol and water into the bottle, then add the essential oils. Shake the bottle vigorously. Let stand overnight in the refrigerator before using.

DIRECTIONS FOR USE

Shake the bottle well before use. Spray in the room (about 3 times for a 160-square-foot room) only when the baby is not there.

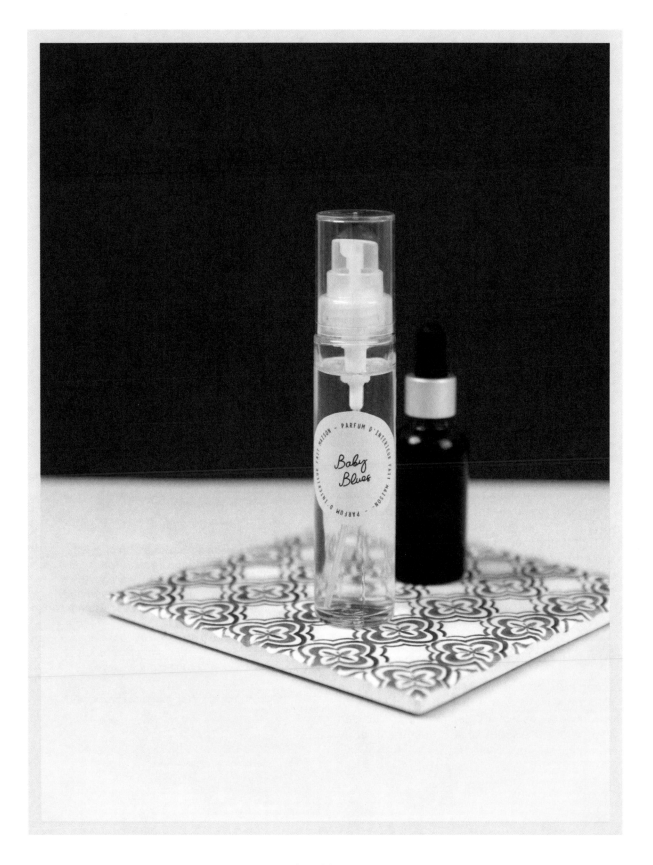

"HYPERSENSITIVITY" AROMATIC SYNERGY BALM

Feeling emotional, crying, mood swings, hypersensitivity, anger, and irritability often result from hormonal changes during and after pregnancy. Some essential oils are wonderful in helping you feel more serene.

Precautions: contains photosensitizing essential oils; avoid sun exposure for 8 hours following application
Preparation time: 15 min
Storage: 12 months
Materials: scale, bowl, pan, spatula
Packaging: 10 ml jar

INGREDIENTS

- 4 g beeswax
- 3 g shea butter
- 3 g sweet almond oil
- 10 drops whole ylang-ylang essential oil
- 10 drops mandarin essence
- 10 drops sweet orange essence

PREPARATION

Combine the beeswax, shea butter, and sweet almond oil in a heat-resistant bowl and melt them in a water bath: fill a saucepan with water, set over low heat, and place the bowl on top of the saucepan. Remove from the heat and stir until the mixture becomes translucent, then add the essential oil and essences and mix quickly. Transfer to the jar before it sets.

DIRECTIONS FOR USE

Scoop out some of the balm and let it melt on your fingers. Massage it into the insides of your wrists, using circular motions. You can also inhale the scent of the mixture directly from your wrists as needed.

TIP

Hypersensitivity is also a sign of great fatigue and built-up stress. Epsom salts provide natural benefits. They are very rich in magnesium sulfate and they warm and soothe the body, allowing muscles and joints to relax for supreme relief. Prepare yourself a relaxing bath by throwing a big handful of salts in the bathtub as the water is running, then relax!

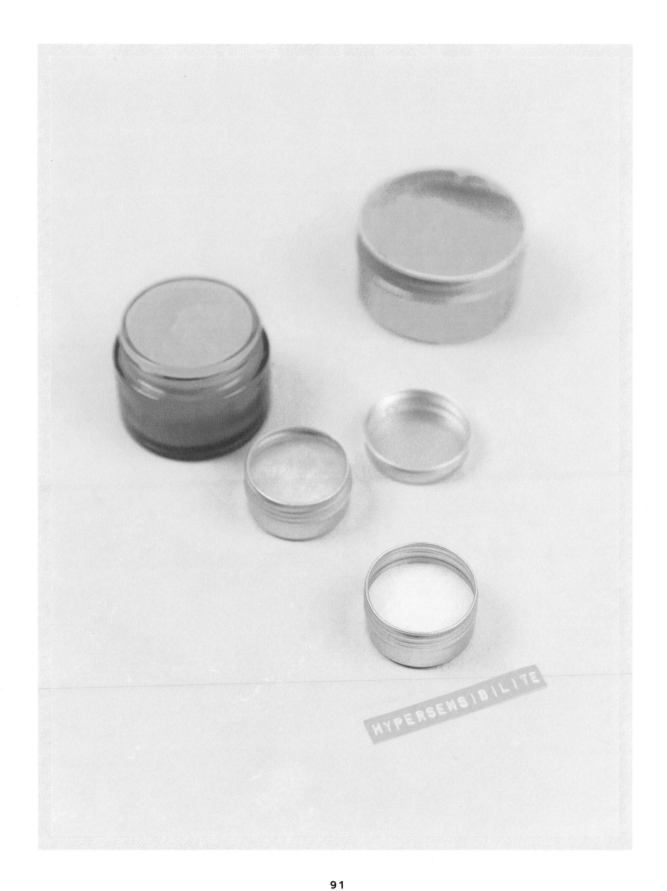

TREATMENTS FOR BABY

BABY'S NEEDS

By Hélène Boyé, naturalist midwife

~~~~~~

Your baby is a little person who expresses his or her needs with body movements, facial expressions, and crying.

Recognizing and understanding a newborn's basic needs is a journey that involves listening, touching, and mothering. There is no absolute dogma for this: every mother is her baby's "specialist" as she pays attention to what she feels and observes.

Everyone can use "I don't know why, but . . ." and "I feel my baby needs . . ." as guides.

Feel like your baby is wanting to sleep? Observe how powerful your voice can be. An Italian study[5] showed that lullabies help strengthen bonding. In addition, the frequency of crying episodes decreases, along with the mother's stress levels.

Babies like to sleep in the living room because domestic noises like the sound of the washing machine and the voices of parents, brothers, and sisters will be reassuring and lull them to sleep. Newborns are very social beings, and silence is not reassuring; on the contrary, they will sleep deeply in a crib placed in the main room while you visit with your friends or relatives.

Your baby needs contact, preferably skin-to-skin.

Cuddle, massage, rock, and carry your baby as often as possible. This allows your baby to secrete oxytocin, the hormone of well-being, bonding, and emotional security. You will also secrete some yourself, and this will foster relaxation as well as milk production. To encourage relaxation and calm, you can massage the soles of your baby's feet or palms, over the pajamas or on the skin, using circular movements in a clockwise direction. This massage can be done when the baby is in need of comfort, is falling asleep, or after a bath.

A baby's essential needs require your physical presence, so opt for babywearing, even in the house. This will allow you to go about your business or be present for your other children while simultaneously caring for your baby.

Baby care should be as simple as possible, since it is now advised to give babies a bath only every two or three days so the skin does not dry out from very hard water. Clean the buttocks with an oleo-calcareous liniment (a milk wash for the skin) you've made yourself and let air-dry as often as possible, or, even better, air-dry in the sun when the weather permits it.

~~~~~~

5   G. Persico, L. Antolini et al., "Maternal Singing of Lullabies during Pregnancy and After Birth: Effects on Mother-Infant Bonding," *Women and Birth*, February 2017.

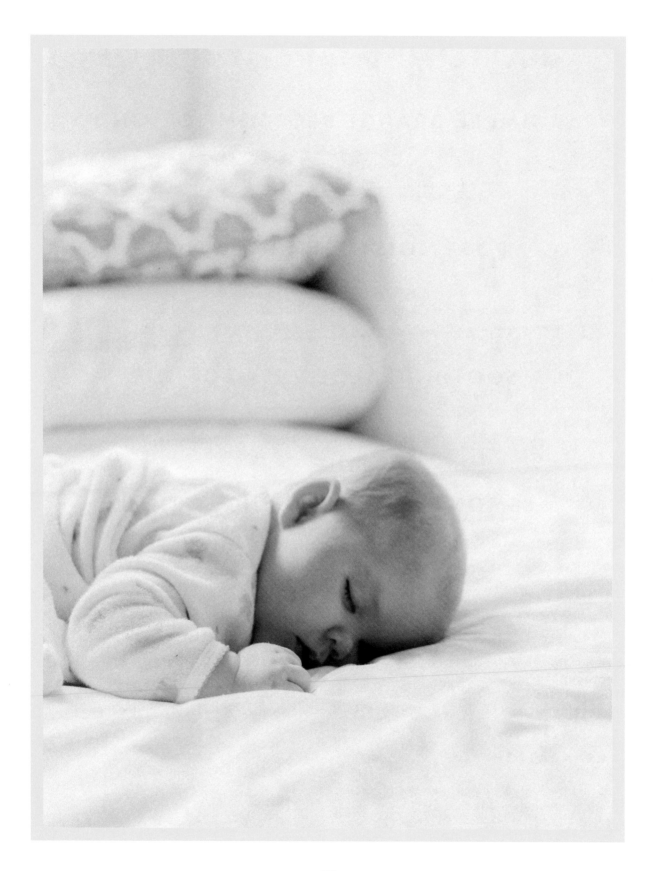

LOTIONS FOR THE FACE

SIMPLE ORANGE BLOSSOM LOTION

100 g spring water, 100 g orange blossom water
(or another hydrosol), 35 drops Cosgard preservative

ROSE MOISTURIZING LOTION

100 g spring water, 75 g rose hydrosol, 15 g vegetable
glycerin, 35 drops Cosgard preservative

SOOTHING ALOE VERA LOTION

130 g spring water, 50 g aloe vera gel, 15 g vegetable
glycerin, 35 drops Cosgard preservative

LEMON BALM CLEANSING LOTION

100 g spring water, 75 g lemon balm hydrosol, 10 g vegetable
glycerin, 10 g jojoba oil, 5 g decyl glucoside surfactant (or an
organic neutral detergent), 35 drops Cosgard preservative

Preparation time: 10 min
Storage: 3 months
Material: scale
Packaging: 200 ml bottle

DIRECTIONS FOR USE

Pour on a washcloth, towelette, or cotton puff,
then clean your baby's face, neck, and hands.

PREPARATION

Pour all the ingredients into the bottle. Close
it and shake it gently to mix well.

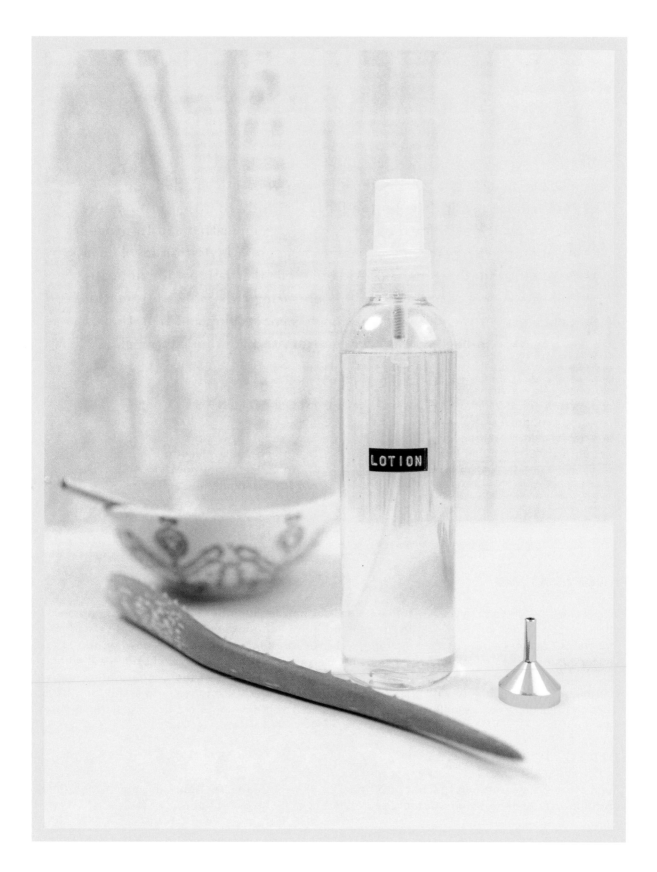

OAT AND CALENDULA CLEANSING MILK

~~~~

Cleansing milk is specially designed to be gentle on delicate skin. Feel free to use it daily on the face, the body, and the bottom. The milk makes it possible to easily remove all impurities and to prevent hypersensitivity reactions by maintaining good hydration levels. Oat is an ultra-soothing and antioxidant agent that is ideal for delicate, sensitive, and reactive skin. This cleansing milk allows for gentle cleansing of the skin without soap, calms itching and irritations, boosts skin healing and regeneration, and soothes atopic skin.

Preparation time: 20 min
Storage: 4 months
Materials: scale, bowl, pan, mini whisk, spatula
Packaging: 100 ml pump bottle

INGREDIENTS

- 55 g spring water
- 8 g vegetable glycerin
- 5 g colloidal oat powder
- 26 g calendula macerated oil
- 4 g vegetable emulsifying wax (Végémulse or Olivem 1000)
- 2 drops natural vitamin E
- 10 drops Cosgard preservative

PREPARATION

Whisk the spring water, glycerin, and colloidal oat powder together in a heat-resistant bowl to obtain a consistent mixture. Add the remaining ingredients except the preservative and melt in a water bath: fill a saucepan with water, set over low heat, and place the bowl on top of the saucepan. Once the emulsifying wax has completely melted, remove the bowl from the heat and, using a whisk, emulsify vigorously until the mixture is opaque. Add the Cosgard preservative and mix for another minute with a spatula. Transfer to the bottle and leave to stand for 2 days, shaking occasionally. The milk will still be liquid, but will develop a creamy consistency after 48 hours.

DIRECTIONS FOR USE

Pump 1 or 2 times on an organic cotton puff or a washable wipe. Apply to your baby's face, bottom, and hands to clean, protect, and moisturize the skin. Do not rinse off.

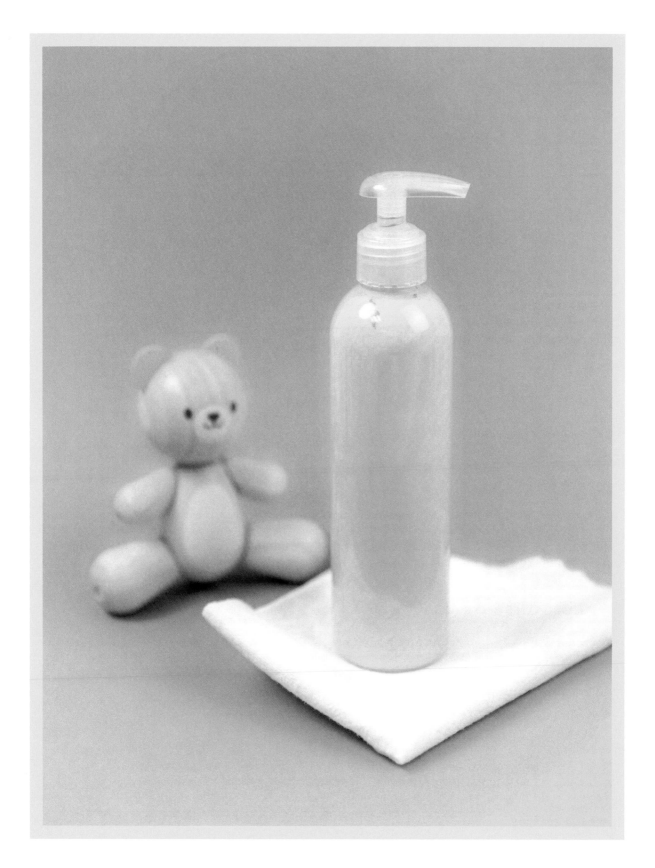

SOS ALL-PURPOSE BALM
FOR NEWBORNS

This rich balm is an optimal treatment for sensitive, dry, or damaged skin. Enriched with calendula macerated oil, it nourishes, soothes, repairs, regenerates, and heals. Its natural formula is vegan and very gentle, and it is suitable for the whole family, especially newborns.

Preparation time: 15 min
Storage: 12 months
Materials: scale, bowl, pan, spatula
Packaging: 50 ml jar

INGREDIENTS

- 5 g candelilla wax
- 15 g shea butter
- 10 g calendula macerated oil
- 10 g oat oil
- 10 g avocado oil
- 2 drops natural vitamin E

PREPARATION

Combine all the ingredients in a heat-resistant bowl and melt in a water bath: fill a saucepan with water, set over very low heat, and place the bowl on top of the saucepan. Remove from the heat, mix for a few seconds with a spatula, and then transfer to the jar. Leave in the refrigerator for 20 minutes to set, then let stand for 12 hours before use.

DIRECTIONS FOR USE

Scoop out some of the balm and let it melt on your fingers. Apply to the affected areas.

TIP

Newborns secrete endorphins (pain-relieving substances) while sucking. Put your baby to your breast for a few minutes to soothe, calm, or lull them to sleep.

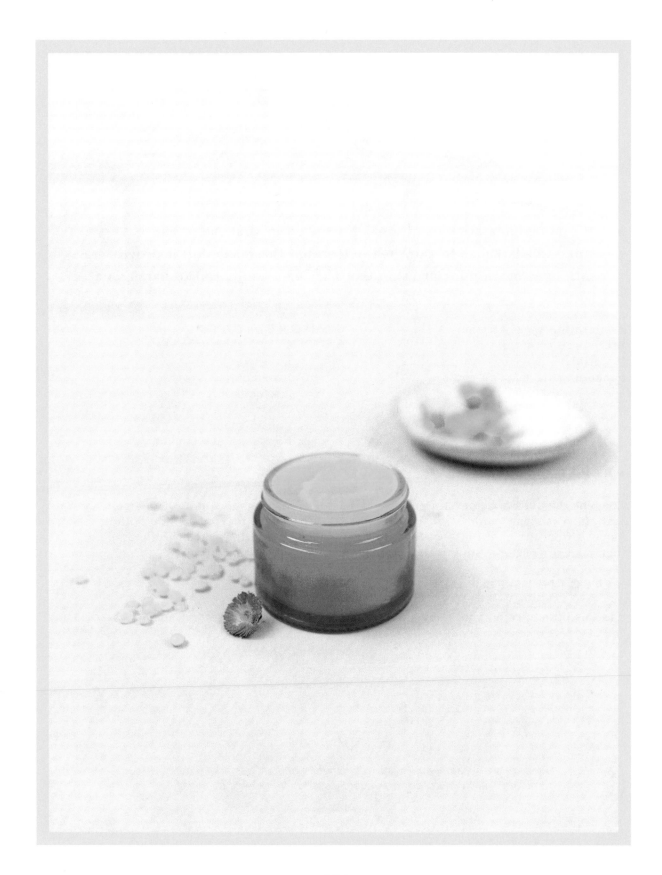

PROTECTIVE WINTER BALM STICK

This gliding stick can be easily stowed in your purse and is very practical! Thanks to the shea butter and the bisabolol, it provides a soothing sensation for dry skin that has been subjected to harsh weather.

Preparation time: 15 min
Storage: 9 months
Materials: scale, bowl, pan, spatula
Packaging: 15 ml stick bottle

INGREDIENTS

* 3 g beeswax
* 5 g shea butter
* 5 g sesame oil
* 1/2 teaspoon arrowroot
* 8 drops bisabolol
* 2 drops natural vitamin E

PREPARATION

Combine the beeswax, shea butter, and sesame oil in a heat-resistant bowl and melt in a water bath: fill a saucepan with water, set over low heat, and place the bowl on top of the saucepan. Remove from the heat, let cool for a few minutes, and add the rest of the ingredients. Stir, then pour the mixture into the stick bottle. Leave to cool in the refrigerator for 30 minutes.

DIRECTIONS FOR USE

Use this little stick on your baby's nose, cheeks, and mouth to protect against the cold. You can also use it on the hands.

DID YOU KNOW?

Bisabolol is a substance with anti-inflammatory and antibacterial properties found naturally in chamomile. It is frequently used in treatments for sensitive skin.

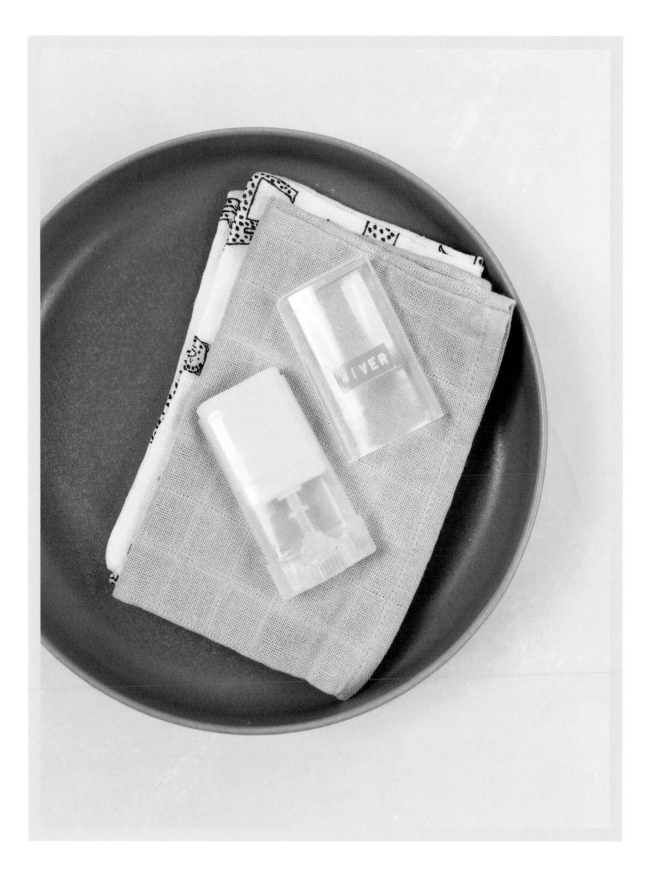

COLD CREAM WITH ORANGE BLOSSOM

~~~~~~~

This is a very useful cold cream to treat skin irritation or dryness. It is highly nourishing and restores the skin's hydrolipidic film, prevents redness, protects from the cold, and is recommended for eczema. A wonderful and versatile care product for the whole family!

Preparation time: 20 min
Storage: 4 months
Materials: scale, bowl, pan, mini whisk
Packaging: 50 ml jar

INGREDIENTS

- 8 g beeswax
- 30 g sweet almond oil
- 12 g orange blossom water
- 10 drops Cosgard preservative

PREPARATION

Combine the beeswax and sweet almond oil in a heat-resistant bowl and melt in a water bath: fill a saucepan with water, set over low heat, and place the bowl on top of the saucepan. When the mixture has a regular consistency, remove from the heat and drizzle in the orange blossom water while emulsifying with a mini-whisk, as if you were making mayonnaise. Add the Cosgard preservative and continue to whisk until it has cooled completely to prevent the mixture from releasing water. Pour into the jar.

DIRECTIONS FOR USE

Scoop out a small amount of cream and apply it with long, massaging movements until it is completely absorbed. This cold cream leaves a slightly oily, occlusive, and protective film on the skin. If water droplets appear on the surface of the cream after a few days, it's nothing serious: just remove them by turning the jar upside down and leaving it over a clean cloth for a few minutes.

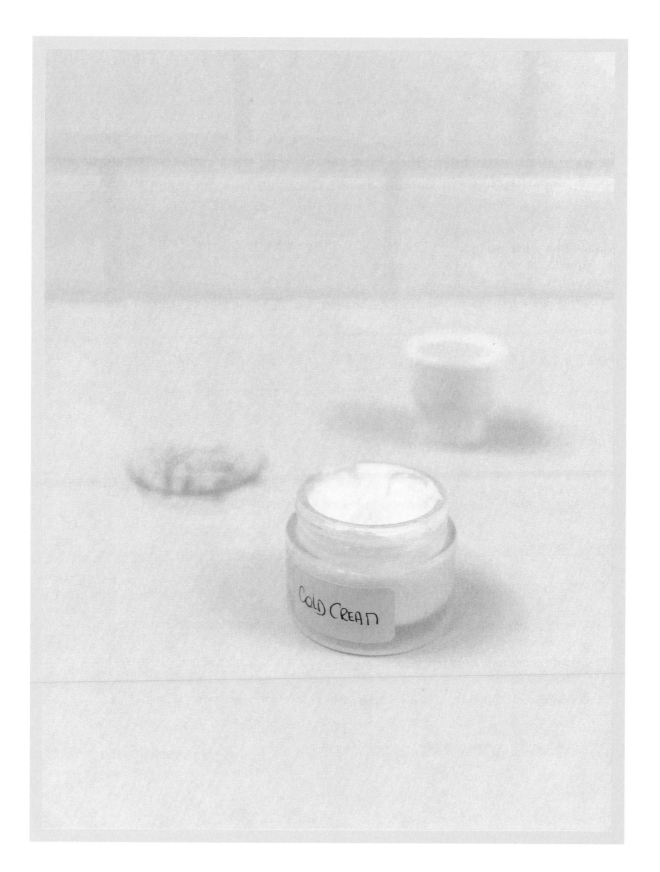

ANTI-CRADLE CAP OIL

~~~

When a baby has "cradle cap," there are small white to yellow patches or scales on the head. They form on the scalp as a result of seborrheic dermatitis and can also appear on the eyebrows and even the face.

Preparation time: 10 min
Storage: 12 months
Material: scale
Packaging: 30 ml tinted glass bottle

INGREDIENTS

* 15 g oat oil
* 15 g calendula macerated oil
* 5 drops natural vitamin E

PREPARATION

Pour the ingredients one by one into the bottle. Close it, then shake it gently.

DIRECTIONS FOR USE

A few hours before bath time, gently massage your child's scalp with a few drops of this mixture, which will loosen the crusts. Don't be afraid to massage this area, even if it is soft—it will not harm the brain. Wash the hair, then style it with a soft brush.

GOOD HABITS

* *Avoid scratching the scaly patches, which can stimulate sebum production and aggravate the problem.*
* *Wash your baby's head with a gentle, sulfate-free product. Rinse well and then gently dry your baby's head.*
* *Brush your baby's hair with a very soft baby hairbrush that is gentle on the scalp.*

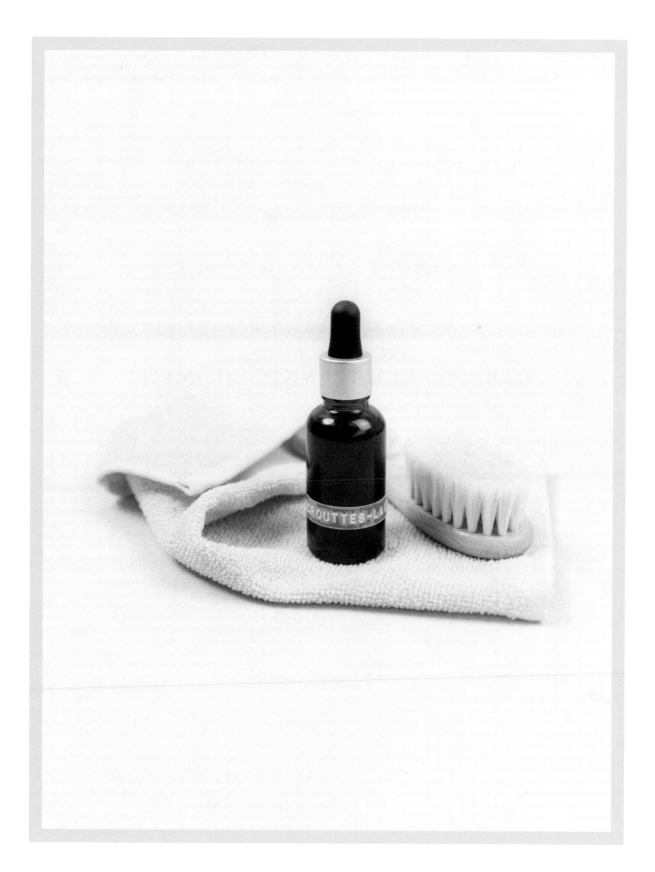

LINIMENTS

A liniment is very easy to make and only has a few ingredients. You can use it to clean as well as protect your baby's bottom. The acidity in the urine and stool is harsh on toddlers' skin, and the liniment maintains the skin's pH while leaving a natural protective film until the next diaper change.

BASIC LINIMENT WITH OLIVE OIL

120 g virgin olive oil, 80 g lime water (available in pharmacies or health food stores)

APRICOT TENDERNESS LINIMENT

80 g apricot oil, 40 g shea butter, 80 g lime water (available in pharmacies or health food stores), 50 drops apricot aromatic extract (optional)

SENSITIVE SKIN LINIMENT

80 g calendula macerated oil, 20 g raspberry oil, 20 g shea butter, 75 g lime water (available in pharmacies or health food stores), 5 g zinc oxide (or white clay)

Preparation time: 10 min
Storage: 6 months
Materials: scale; food processor *or* salad bowl and hand blender
Packaging: 200 ml pump bottle

PREPARATION

Blend all ingredients for several minutes, until you obtain a milk that is stable and uniform. Pour into the pump bottle.

DIRECTIONS FOR USE

Pump out the liniment once or twice on an organic cotton puff or a washable wipe and apply it to the buttocks, always starting from the base to the top.

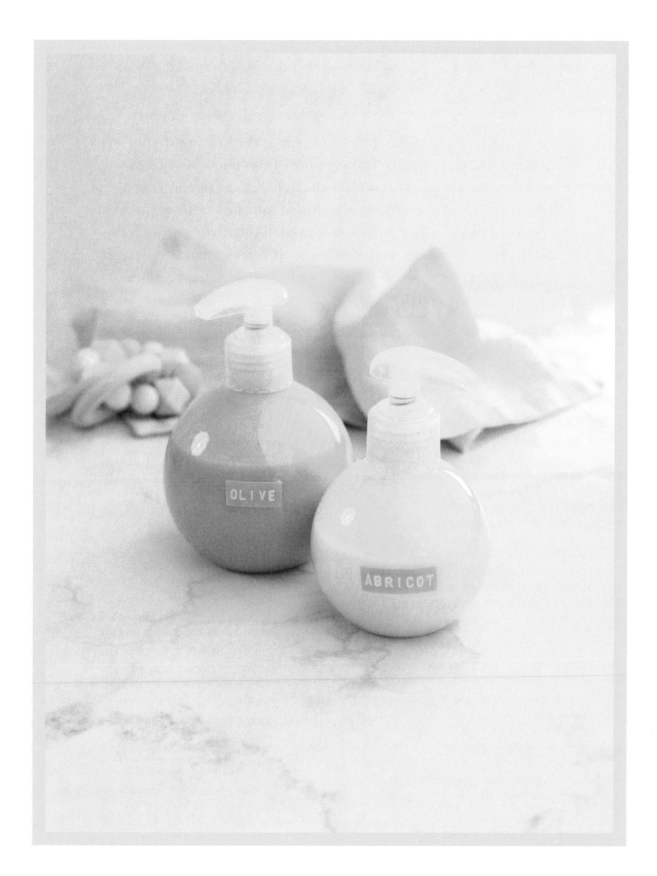

DIAPER-CHANGING BALM

Diaper rash is when the baby's skin is irritated in the diaper area. This can result in simple redness or, in the most severe cases, bleeding and skin abrasions. Conventional diapers can cause this because they retain moisture and heat and don't allow the skin to breathe. All it takes is this melting balm to soothe the baby's irritated skin during a diaper change. It forms an anti-moisture barrier, softens, moisturizes, and prevents diaper rash.

Preparation time: 15 min
Storage: 9 months
Materials: scale, bowl, pan, mini whisk
Packaging: 50 ml jar

INGREDIENTS

- 5 g zinc oxide (or calamine)
- 5 g spring water
- 25 g shea butter
- 15 g rose hip oil
- 5 g beeswax
- 1 drop natural vitamin E

PREPARATION

Mix the zinc oxide with the spring water in a heat-resistant bowl using a mini whisk. Once you've obtained a uniform white paste, add the rest of the ingredients, then make a water bath: fill a saucepan with water, set over low heat, and place the bowl on top of the saucepan. When the beeswax is melted, remove from the heat, mix vigorously, and pour the mixture into the jar. Place in the refrigerator for 30 minutes. Let stand at room temperature for 12 hours before use.

DIRECTIONS FOR USE

Take a dab of balm and use it to massage the irritated areas of the bottom. There's no need to rub the balm in deeply: a thin layer is enough to provide protective benefits. This zinc balm also soothes and dries the small seeping sores that the baby may have on the buttocks, thighs, neck, or in the folds of the skin.

GOOD HABITS

- *In the event of erythema, check your baby's diaper regularly and change it as soon as it's dirty.*

- *Clean your baby's bottom with soapy water and thoroughly dry the skin before putting on the diaper.*

- *Let your baby go diaper-free for a few hours, with the buttocks exposed to the air.*

- *Apply a thick layer of zinc oxide treatment.*

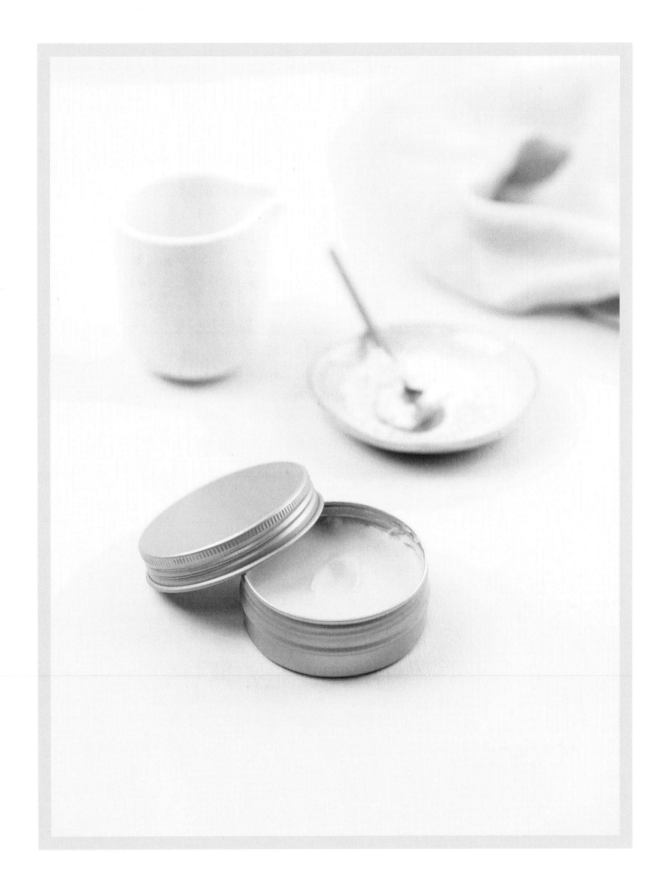

VEGETAL RICE TALC WITH LAVENDER

Most of the powders on the market today are talc-based. Used by most women in their makeup or for their baby, talc is now controversial because its quality is inconsistent. It can contain traces of asbestos or useless, sometimes even allergenic, additives. Talc is not irritating to the skin, but it should not be applied to wounds; it is therefore contraindicated if your baby has severe erythema. In homemade formulas, it can be replaced by starches or micronized precooked flours, which are very soft and absorbent. Corn starch, oat or rice cream, and arrowroot or white clay soften, absorb moisture, and create a protective film between the diaper and the skin. This powder, with a base of rice cream and sweet almond oil, can replace most commercially available talcum powders. It absorbs moisture and leaves the skin soft. It is recommended for protecting the baby's buttocks after each diaper change because it leaves a film that soothes and provides light insulation.

Preparation time: 15 min
Storage: 12 months
Materials: scale, mortar, pestle
Packaging: 200 g jar with a small sieve

INGREDIENTS

- 70 g rice cream powder
- 15 g white clay
- 5 g zinc oxide
- 1 drop true lavender essential oil (Lavandula officinalis)
- 5 drops sweet almond oil

PREPARATION

In a mortar, work the powders, essential oil, and sweet almond oil with a pestle until a consistent powder is obtained, without lumps. Put it in a jar with a small sieve.

DIRECTIONS FOR USE

After changing the diaper, powder your baby's clean, dry bottom with this soft powder.

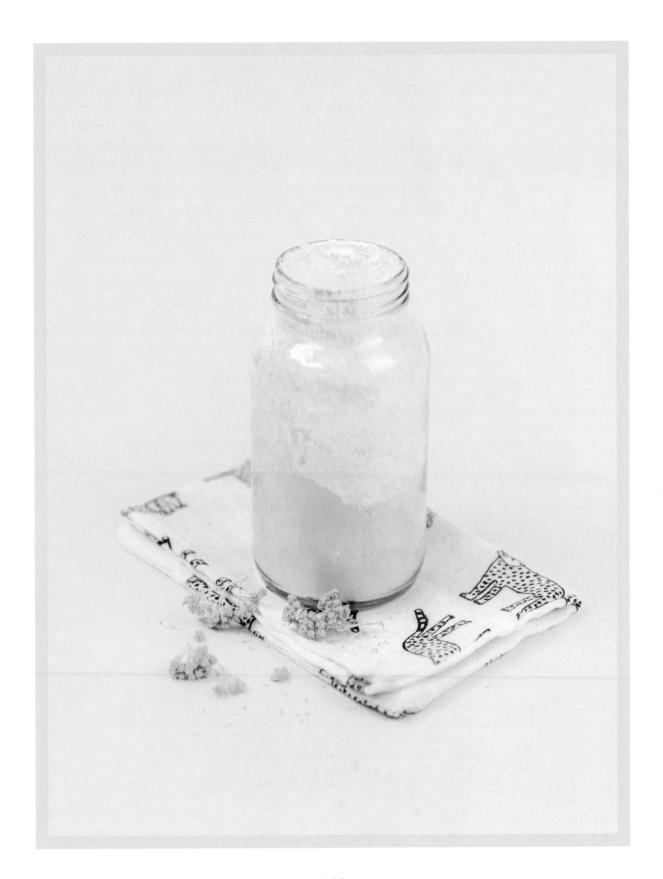

MASSAGE OIL

One of the first senses acquired in utero is touch. While in your belly, your baby was massaged by and could perceive your movements. Bringing these sensations back to life through massage restores this reassuring relationship for your baby. In certain cultures, it is common to practice baby massage. It calms, improves sleep, and relieves digestive problems like colic and constipation. Squalane is one of the components of the sebum that our skin secretes naturally; it is also present in certain plants such as olives. It is a fluid and silky oil that protects the skin and restores the natural lipid barrier. You can also opt for jojoba oil, which is soft and balancing.

Preparation time: 5 min
Storage: 9 months
Material: scale
Packaging: 30 ml bottle

INGREDIENTS

- 10 g vegetable squalane (or jojoba oil)
- 10 g apricot oil
- 10 g calendula macerated oil

PREPARATION

Pour the ingredients one by one into the bottle. Close it, then shake it gently to mix the oils well.

DIRECTIONS FOR USE

Take the equivalent of a 1/2 teaspoon of oil into your hand. Warm it for a few seconds between your palms, then perform the massage.

GOOD HABITS

- *Set up your space in a warm room with soft light.*
- *Be sure to choose a safe place where your child won't fall.*
- *Wash your hands well and warm them up if necessary.*
- *Remove jewelry and watches to avoid hurting your baby.*
- *Turn off your phone, television, or radio, or put on soft music.*
- *Avoid massaging your baby after breastfeeding or bottle feeding.*

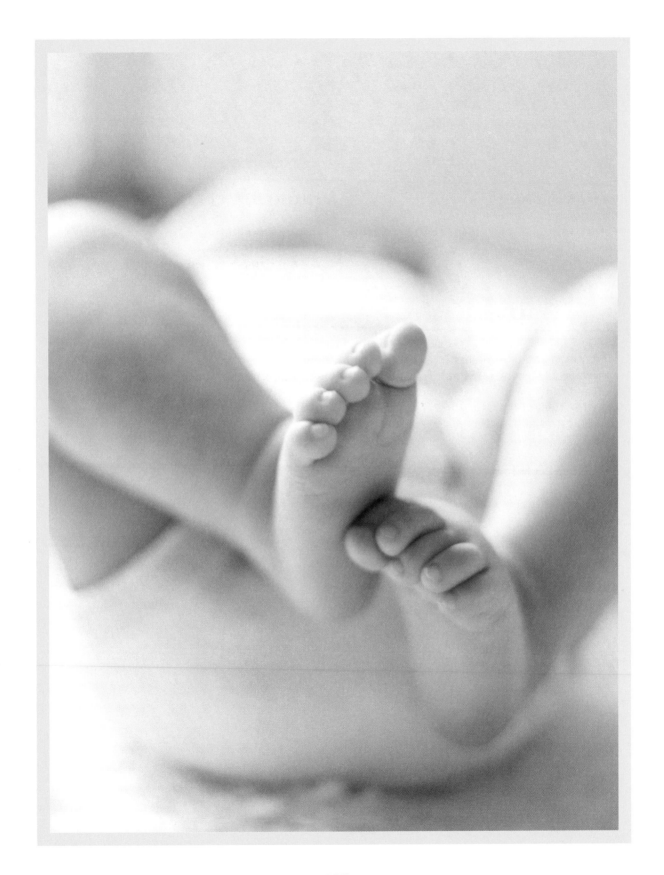

CALENDULA MASSAGE BAR

~~~~~~~~

Preparation time: 10 min
Storage: 3 months
Materials: scale, bowl, pan, spatula, silicone mold (50 g capacity)
Packaging: none

INGREDIENTS

- 16 g shea butter
- 16 g candelilla wax
- 16 g calendula macerated oil
- 2 g arrowroot (optional)
- 4 drops natural vitamin E

PREPARATION

Combine all the ingredients in a heat-resistant bowl and melt in a water bath: fill a saucepan with water, set over low heat, and place the bowl on top of the saucepan. Remove from the heat and stir until the mixture becomes translucent, then pour it quickly into the mold. Leave to set in the refrigerator for 2 hours. Turn out of the mold and let stand for 1 day at room temperature before use.

DIRECTIONS FOR USE

Warm the bar between your hands until it leaves a creamy oil, then perform the massage.

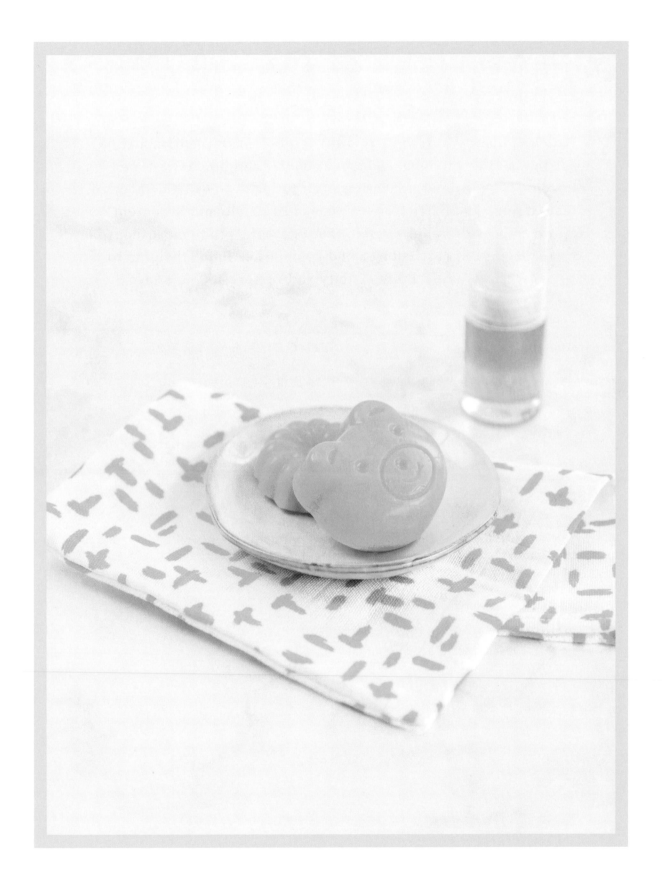

ANTI-ECZEMA BALM

Rich in omega-3, raspberry oil is a powerful anti-inflammatory that soothes itching, reduces redness, and boosts skin cell regeneration. It is particularly suited to highly sensitive, reactive, and atopic skin. Safflower oil, thanks to its vitamin K content, is known to provide relief for skin that is atopic-prone or susceptible to redness. It restructures and replenishes lipids, helping to preserve the skin's elasticity and restore its moisture.

Preparation time: 20 min
Storage: 9 months
Materials: scale, bowl, pan, mini whisk
Packaging: 50 ml jar

INGREDIENTS

- 10 g candelilla wax
- 10 g shea butter
- 10 g safflower oil
- 10 g raspberry oil
- 10 g calendula macerated oil
- 5 drops natural vitamin E

PREPARATION

Combine all the ingredients in a heat-resistant bowl and melt in a water bath: fill a saucepan with water, set over low heat, and place the bowl on top of the saucepan. Remove from the heat and stir until the mixture becomes translucent. Transfer to the pot. Leave to cool in the refrigerator for 20 minutes, then let stand for 12 hours before use.

DIRECTIONS FOR USE

Use this balm to massage the affected areas 2 or 3 times a day.

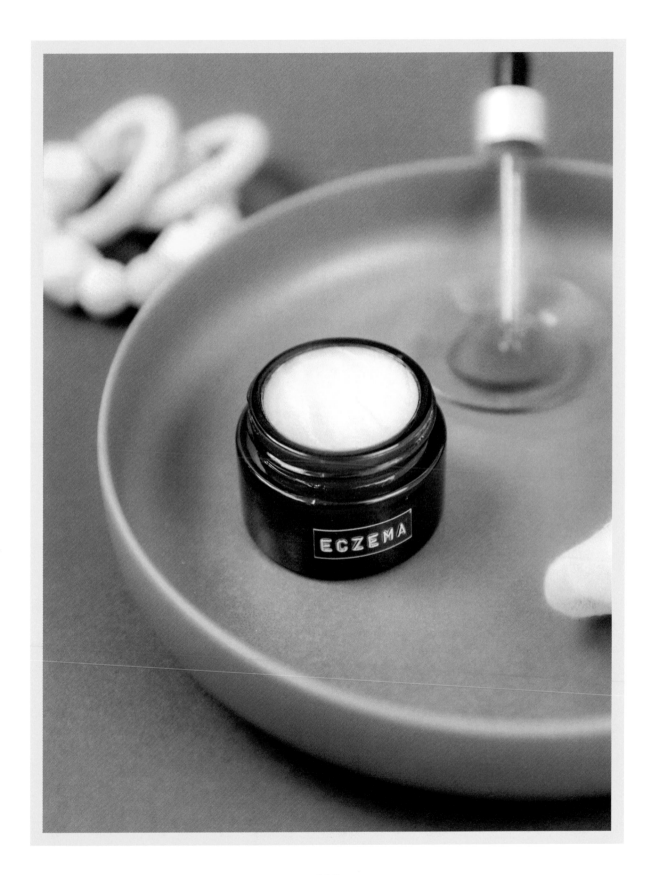

FOAMING BATH CLEANSER

Bath time is very special and a real source of enjoyment. Knowing that a baby's skin is thin and therefore sensitive to chemical agents until about four years of age, and also that skin is 20 percent more absorbent when wet, makes it clear why it is essential to choose natural and specialized care products. Don't just make your choices blindly! Conventional shower gels, even those specially formulated for babies, are loaded with irritating, sometimes toxic, substances. This cleaner uses soap nuts. The soap nut is the fruit of the soap nut tree, which grows in Kashmir. Its shell is filled with saponin, which dissolves when it comes in contact with water to release a soft and powerful soap. It can be used as a body and hair cleanser as well as a 100 percent natural detergent.

Preparation time: 20 min
Storage: 3 months
Materials: scale, pan, spatula, coffee filter, funnel, salad bowl
Packaging: 250 ml foam bottle

INGREDIENTS

- 250 g spring water
- 1 large handful soap nuts (7 to 8 nuts)
- 20 g vegetable glycerin
- 20 g sweet almond oil
- 40 drops Cosgard preservative

PREPARATION

In a saucepan, bring the spring water and soap nuts to a boil. Turn down the heat to the lowest setting and simmer for 5 minutes. Turn off the heat and let cool. Set a coffee filter inside a funnel and filter the mixture into a bowl to remove the particles of soap nuts. Then add the rest of the ingredients and pour into the bottle.

DIRECTIONS FOR USE

Use this mousse instead of your baby's shower gel to clean the face, hair, and body.

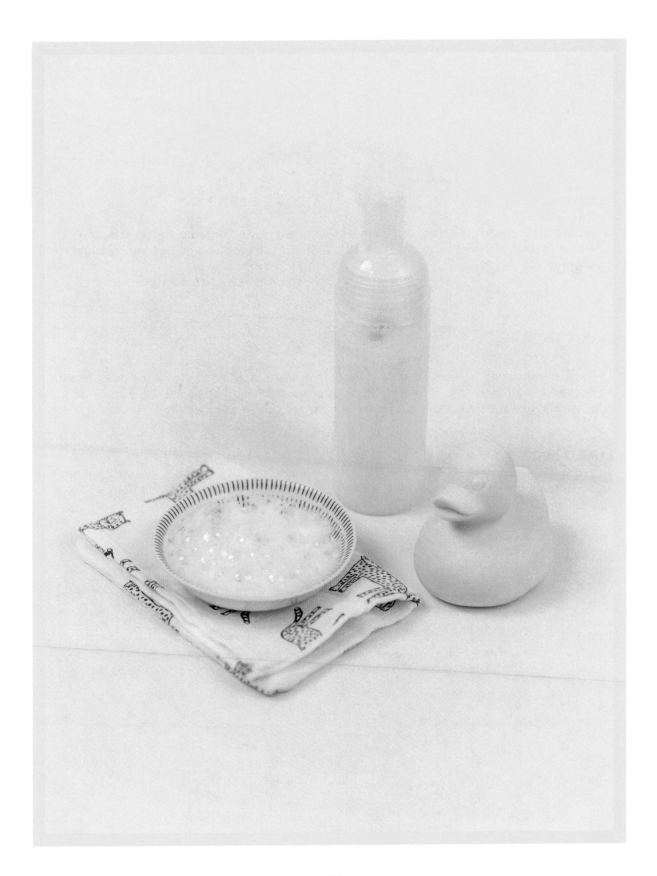

AVOCADO SOAP CREAM

~~~~~~

Preparation time: 20 min
Storage: 3 months
Materials: scale, salad bowl and hand blender or food processor, spatula
Packaging: 250 ml jar

INGREDIENTS

* 25 g grated organic Marseille soap
* 200 g boiled and cooled spring water
* 20 g avocado oil
* 40 drops Cosgard preservative

PREPARATION

Put the Marseille soap and boiled spring water in a large salad bowl. Work the mixture with a hand blender until there are no more pieces of soap. Add the rest of the ingredients and mix for a few minutes with a spatula to remove the last of the air bubbles. Pour into the jar.

DIRECTIONS FOR USE

Use this cream instead of your baby's shower gel to clean the face, hair, and body.

GOOD HABITS

* *Choose organic cleaning bases specially formulated for babies.*

* *Check the INCI ingredient list for sulfates and PEGs.*

* *If you decide on a solid soap, choose one that is cold saponified (CS) and superfatted. It is gentler on the skin and does not alter the natural hydrolipidic film.*

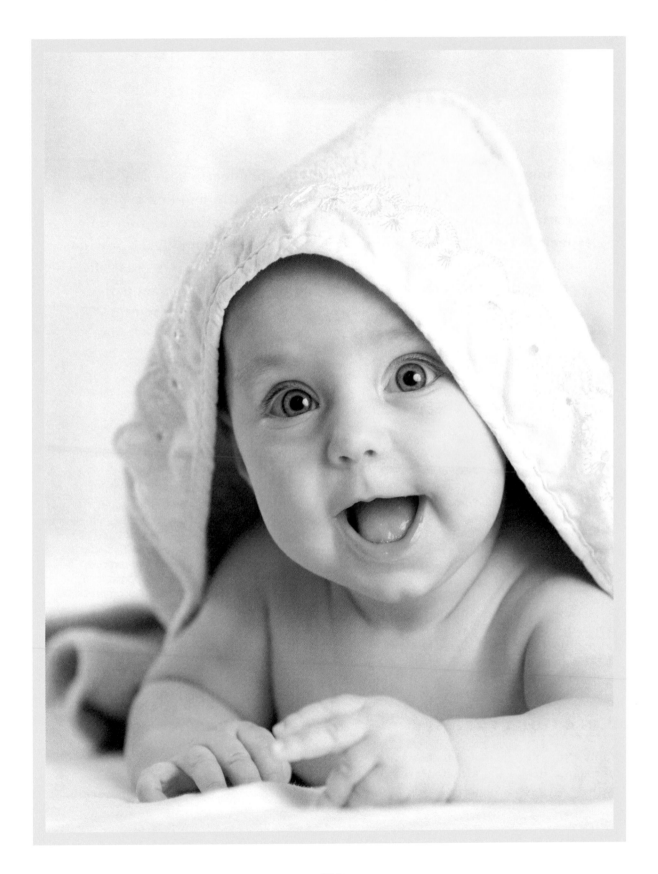

ARNICA TREATMENT
BALM FOR BUMPS AND BRUISES

~~~

As soon as a baby begins to be more independent, especially when learning to walk, there are many risks. Your little budding explorer is attracted to everything within reach, and it's a time for you to be especially vigilant. The mountain arnica (Arnica montana) plant provides quick relief in the event of a fall, bump, or bruise. It is a great ally for mothers, both as an ointment and in the form of homeopathic granules. This remedy is only effective on superficial injuries.

Preparation time: 10 min
Storage: 12 months
Materials: scale, bowl, pan, spatula
Packaging: 50 ml jar

INGREDIENTS

* 10 g beeswax
* 30 g arnica macerated oil
* 10 g tamanu oil
* 2 drops natural vitamin E

PREPARATION

Combine all the ingredients in a bowl and melt in a water bath: fill a saucepan with water, set over low heat, and place the bowl on top of the saucepan. Remove from the heat, mix gently with a spatula, then transfer to the pot.

DIRECTIONS FOR USE

Apply the ointment several times a day by massaging it into the affected area. Do not apply to an open wound.

GOOD HABITS

* *For a simple bump, to help minimize the bruise, apply a cold washcloth or an ice bag for about 10 minutes.*

* *After a fall, your baby may suffer from a cut or compromised skin. If the wound is only superficial, you can treat it at home. Clean it with soapy water and use tweezers to remove any small pieces. Then apply a local disinfectant using a sterile compress. Protect the wound with a dressing made out of honey, which will allow it to heal in the open air. Honey has always been part of the popular pharmacopoeia; it is used to treat boils, ulcers, and wounds of all kinds. It is antibacterial and helps with scar formation, and therefore speeds up the healing process.*

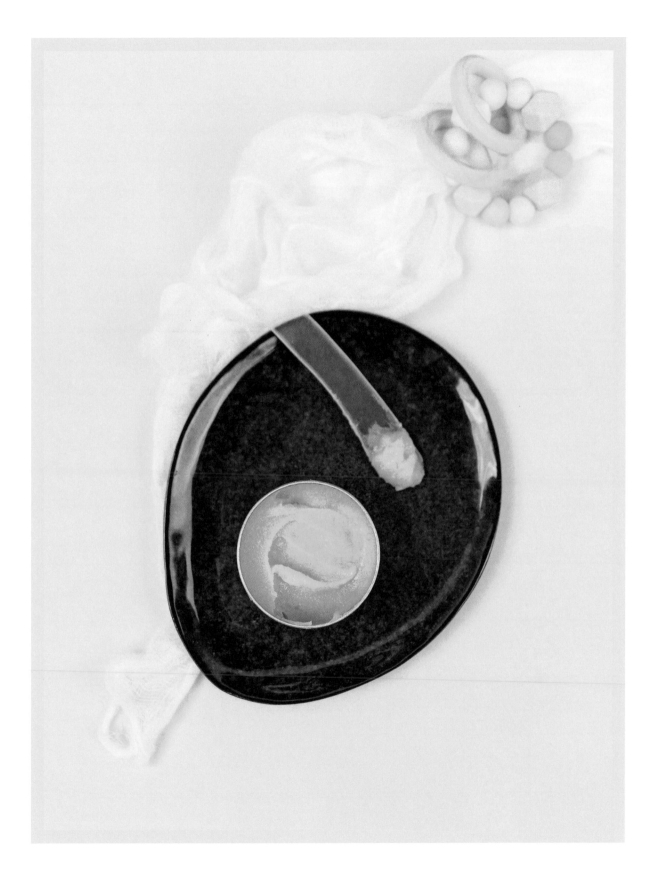

PLANT OILS

Normal skin	Jojoba, sweet almond, apricot, camellia
Combination to oily skin	Jojoba, calendula, hazelnut, macadamia, melon, camellia, white tea
Dry, dehydrated, alipidic skin	Apricot, avocado, sweet almond, wheat germ, olive, evening primrose, argan
Mature or damaged skin	Jojoba, cranberry, rose hip, argan, apple seed, raspberry, black cumin, calendula macerated oil
Sensitive baby skin	Jojoba, avocado, oat, raspberry, calendula macerated oil

AROMATIC HYDROSOLS

Normal skin	Rose, fine lavender, orange blossom (neroli), bamboo
Combination to oily skin	Geranium bourbon, lemon, fine lavender, tea tree, bamboo, white willow
Dry, dehydrated, alipidic skin	Orange blossom (neroli), sambac jasmine, sandalwood
Mature or damaged skins	Wild carrot, ladaniferus rockrose, witch hazel, sandalwood
Sensitive baby skin	Rose, orange blossom (neroli), lemon balm, fine lavender

RESOURCES

~~~~~~~~~~

RAW MATERIALS FOR COSMETICS

Aroma-Zone: www.aroma-zone.com
Make It Beauty: www.make-it-beauty.com
Huiles & Sens: www.huiles-et-sens.com/fr
Labo Hévéa: http://en.labo-hevea.com
Joli Essence: www.joliessence.com
My Cosmetik: www.mycosmetik.fr
Bilby & Co: www.bilby-co.com
Herboristerie du Palais-Royal: www.herboristerie.com

GOOD TIPS FOR FUTURE MOMS AND BABIES

Eco-friendly wipes for moms and babies:
www.tendances-emma.fr

100 percent latex toys hand-painted in Barcelona:
https://oliandcarol.us

A Scandinavian slow living brand, including pretty wooden rattles:
www.liewood.com

A superb selection of green and environmentally committed designers:
https://smallable.com/page/greenable

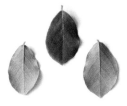